ADD on the Job

ALSO BY LYNN WEISS:

Attention Deficit Disorder in Adults
The Attention Deficit Disorder in Adults Workbook
Power Lines (coauthor)

ADD on the Job

Making Your ADD Work for You

Dr. Lynn Weiss

Taylor Publishing Company
Dallas, Texas

6125348

Published by Taylor Publishing Company
1550 West Mockingbird Lane
Dallas, Texas 75235

Library of Congress Cataloging-in-Publication Data

Weiss, Lynn.
ADD on the job : making your ADD work for you / Lynn Weiss.
p.   cm.
Includes index.
ISBN 0-87833-917-5
1. Vocational guidance. 2. Attention-deficit disordered adults—
Employment. 3. Job stress. 4. Interpersonal communication.
5. Time management. 6. Career changes. I. Title.
HF5381.W4344   1996
650.1'087—dc20
                                                              95-47458
                                                                  CIP

Printed in the United States of America

10 9 8 7 6 5 4 3 2 1

Table of Contents

Acknowledgments

Many people contributed to the completion of this book. Those with ADD who told their stories to me wanted them passed on to others. Their kindness and willingness to mentor others dealing with being ADD is heartfelt. Thanks for the caring.

Janis Dworkis, who helped me structure this book, deserves my greatest praise. As we learned to understand each other's way of looking at the world and expressing ourselves, we learned more about ourselves—and I learned more about ADD than I knew before. I've passed on what I learned to you in these pages.

Mary Kelly, my agent, per usual, held a belief in the importance of communicating about ADD. With her support and motivation, I tackled this project. With her unflagging encouragement, I continue to live my dreams. Thank you.

Many thanks also to Mary Schultz, the Comma Queen, who let me take over her dining room table as every word was read aloud and every phrase, sentence, and paragraph were checked.

My appreciation to Holly McGuire, my editor at Taylor, and Anita Edson, Taylor's publicist, who, with all the other wonderful Taylor people, are responsible for getting this book in the hands of those who can use it.

And finally, thanks to everyone who supported and believed in this project. The teamwork paid off.

1

About ADD

I am so glad I am ADD!

Are you surprised? You might be, if you have always associated ADD with problems, with limits, and with difficulties.

But that's not the way I look at it. The way I see it, I possess special skills and strengths because of ADD, and with those skills I have been able to experience life in Technicolor. I've known diversity, drama, creativity, and sensitivity—all as a result of my ADD. I've had lots of experiences because of it, learned many lessons, and led a rich life.

Let me tell you a little bit about myself, so you'll understand why I wrote this book and what I hope it will do for you.

My official diagnosis of ADD—attention deficit disorder—came only a few years ago. Looking back over my life and careers, I see that even before I knew I had ADD, I was making adjustments for it. For example, during most of the thirty years I spent as a psychotherapist, I used a rocking chair for my office chair. I rocked and rocked, moving constantly. Though I didn't realize it at the time, my hyperactivity was soothed by my rocking, while the people I counseled also felt soothed and nurtured.

In general, when I followed my heart—whether that was rocking in a chair or working with my hands—I was happy being me.

Unfortunately, there were many times I did not take that path. Instead, I did what I thought was expected of me, which in most instances did not fit my ADD nature. I tried to learn things the way I was taught to learn them. I stayed in school. Although not performing up to the level of my intelligence, I managed to be successful. This meant that I struggled to follow a path that often ignored my creative way of thinking, learning, and doing things. The tangible result of my struggles was earning the academic degrees that allowed me to counsel people and gain the opportunity to have others listen to me. The emotional result was depression.

But I was aided along my path by a psychiatrist who told me in my twenties, "Lynn, trust your feelings. You are sensitive, and they will guide you."

What he really did was give me permission to trust my feelings. I did, and that became the strongest tool of my life. When I follow my heart and trust my feelings, I experience success and happiness.

It all boils down to being who I am. And that approach goes for everyone. Be who you are—however and whoever that is.

Over the years, I have learned both to listen within myself to understand my true feelings and to watch the external world outside of myself to understand what is expected of me. It then becomes my job and my responsibility to merge those two aspects of life—the way I feel and what the world expects of me—without losing any of myself in the process.

As a young adult I couldn't decide whether I wanted to be an artist or a psychotherapist. Finally one day while in New York City, sculpting a Madonna-like figure out of clay, the proverbial light bulb went off in my head, and the decision was made: I wanted to help people more than make things. In retrospect, I see I wanted to find answers for myself, of course, but I didn't need to know that then. What I did need to know was that I wanted people and our humanness to be the focus of my life.

Every choice I made to prepare myself to work as a psychotherapist was different from standard operating procedure, different from the way other people were doing things. For example, I didn't major in psychology or medicine because I wasn't able to read well enough or retain facts well enough to be successful in those areas. Instead, I sought a master's degree in anthropology with an emphasis on psychiatric anthropology. In the long run, anthropology and its main research technique of participant observation turned out to be the best teacher I could have found, the best teacher for me given the way my brain works (ADD) and what I wanted to achieve.

I was in graduate school in the 1960s, a time of great experimentation in many fields. In education many unusual programs existed. For example, the National Institute of Mental Health offered predoctoral anthropology students a clinical internship at the University of Washington Medical School's Department of Psychiatry. The idea was to train anthropologists to do quality psychiatric field work in various cultures. The program was wonderful for me. I received excellent clinical training and, in fact, have used it ever since: doing clinical work from the broad perspective that anthropology's participant observation methods make possible.

Next I spent time in the community taking mental health care into homes, schools, and workplaces. With experience in hand, I then began a long career in counseling, bolstered by a Ph.D. in multidisciplinary studies with an emphasis in child development and affective education. What a wonderfully creative focus for someone who has ADD! During my years of counseling, I saw it all: the inside and outside of institutions, individuals and families, couples, children, adolescents and adults, businesses, agencies, and organizations. As I plied my trade, I kept observing, learning, trying new approaches, and noting the results.

That's how ADD surfaced as a focal point in my life. My initial interest in ADD came when my son was diagnosed with it in elementary school. I developed broader interest when I observed that he went through puberty with his ADD intact, even though professionals had always taught that ADD "went away at puberty."

Around the same time that I realized my teenage son was still dealing with his ADD, I noticed that two adults I was counseling had characteristics of ADD. I reasoned that ADD could explain why they weren't yielding to counseling for emotional problems and why they had the problems in the first place—even though everyone "knew" that adults could not have ADD. By changing how I interacted with these clients, I studied the effects that ADD has on a person's behavior and feelings, and I learned that adults *can* have ADD.

Meanwhile, I had become involved in the broadcast business, which turned out to be a wonderful fit for my ADD nature. I began a ten-year period as a radio talk show host, three hours a day, five days a week. During four of those years, I also worked regularly as a TV commentator.

"Have mouth, will travel" became my motto. I had done a lot of public speaking during the previous years, and broadcasting was an extension of that. Even more appealing, the "high" of being on the air and the spontaneity of being asked questions with only three minutes to answer thrilled me. I loved it, and I was successful at it.

During those years, I often heard people say, "I don't know how you do it. You have so much energy. You're so enthusiastic, sensitive, and empathetic." In retrospect, I see that every one of those comments and compliments related directly to my ADD. The particular way in which my brain worked, my ADD, fueled my performances and empowered me.

One day in the mid-1980s, I mentioned on the air that ADD continues into adulthood. Suddenly, the phone lines lit up, and the station switchboard became jammed with calls.

The concept of ADD in adulthood was up and running—and it hasn't stopped yet.

My involvement with ADD during the past ten years has brought me into contact with many wonderful people. I've learned what ADD is and what it's not. And for me, the crowning glory came some eight years after I began working with ADD: that's when I finally recognized that I am ADD.

I had coped with it so well, had so many other explanations for the problems I faced, and had worked so hard to do the things I thought I "should" be able to do—things that were so difficult because of my ADD—that when the veil lifted, I cannot tell you the relief I felt.

Like everyone else who discovers they have ADD, I went through a grieving period. I felt grief for the person who had worked so hard, felt so guilty and ashamed because of inadequacies, carried sadness because of the discrepancy between her potential and her ability to achieve in "acceptable" ways, and for the lost years of trying to be something she was not.

Now joy fills me as I am more and more able to be the person I was always meant to be and as I communicate to others that message of self-acceptance.

I am excited about helping all of us build bridges to one another so that we can utilize our talents fully to solve problems and make the world a better place. Honoring our differences is what this is all about.

What Is ADD?

What neuroscience has shown us recently is that ADD is a distinctive "flavor," or style of brain organization, one that favors creativity and simultaneous multilevel processing over linear, detail-oriented thought. ADD is rooted in biology and neurology, being a genetic trait that was passed to you by one or both of your parents, just like the color of your hair or an artistic talent. You have no more control over the fact that you have ADD than you have over your height or the color of your eyes.

The ways in which ADD has been described and accepted by society has changed a great deal through time. Centuries ago, less emphasis was put on individuals to conform to "structured" settings, and more natural opportunities existed for people with ADD wiring to have places in their society—places of honor, where their skills were valued. As civilization took a more technical direction, people with less ADD, and more linear, brain wiring began to have increased opportunities to gain power and control. Systems developed, organization of all sorts of things blossomed, and the need to pay attention to details and bits and pieces of information took over.

Educational systems replaced educational opportunities and hands-on apprenticeships, and more emphasis was put on learning *about* things than on learning *by doing* things. This approach favored linear wiring, so the schism widened between people with more ADD traits and those whose brains were wired in a more detail-oriented way.

Soon judgments became attached to those differences, judgments leveled by those who built the systems, fit into the systems, and saw anyone who was different as *wrong*. At first, labels with moral implications were placed on those who weren't able to behave in the restrained, focused way of the systems' builders: *lazy, uncaring,* or *bad.*

As our understanding of human behavior progressed, a medically based labeling process took over. Those who were different acquired a label denoting a *disorder*. It wasn't their fault, scientists said. They weren't acting lazy or uncaring on purpose: they had a medical disorder. Thus the term attention deficit *disorder* emerged. In the most recent edition of the American Psychiatric Association's *Diagnostic and Statistical Manual*, ADD, as it pertains to adults, is listed as "attention deficit/hyperactivity disorder" (ADHD), which can further indicate whether the ADD is accompanied by hyperactivity and impulsivity.

But a delay always exists between the clinical understanding of a "condition" and the publication of professional manuals. Concepts will continue to evolve as a better understanding of ADD emerges.

How I See ADD

The more I've come to understand ADD—both through my research into the scientific literature and through my own work with clients—the more I see it as an alternate and perfectly natural way of brain wiring.

Consequently, I believe that an appropriate model for ADD is a continuum—a continuum of human behavior with lots of ADD traits on one end and few or none on the other. I don't see any one particular point on this continuum at which someone suddenly *has* ADD. Rather, I see that individuals have either more or fewer ADD traits, which make it harder or easier for the individual to accomplish certain tasks or perform in certain ways. ADD creates strengths and weaknesses relative to the areas in which an individual is functioning and the expectations placed upon that person.

This way of thinking leaves no room for the term *normal* and no room for identifying a high level of ADD traits as a *disorder*.

Look at it like this: Suppose we took a large group of people and lined them up according to their eye color, from the deepest brown/black to the palest blue. In looking over the whole group, we accept the fact that brown eyes are natural for some people, and green or blue eyes are natural for others. We wouldn't think of saying that brown-eyed people are normal, and blue-eyed people have an "eye-color disorder." But that's exactly what we do when we say that people with a low level of ADD traits are normal, and those with a high level of such traits have a disorder. Let's remember that some people have hazel eyes, just as people can have some ADD traits and some non-ADD traits.

Although I disagree with the labeling of ADD traits as a *disorder*, I will continue to use the term ADD in this book, since it is in such common usage today. But I do not believe that ADD is something you *have*, like a virus or a disease. I believe ADD is something you *are*, just like you are athletic, musical, or tall. So I will use the term *having ADD* throughout this book because that is the common usage, but you will also see the term *being ADD* because that is my deepest belief.

I am not trying to convince you that being ADD-wired is completely wonderful or all fun and games. The truth is—and you and I both know this from personal experience—ADD traits can cause you trouble. *But that does not mean there is something wrong with you.* What it means is that the way you are wired may not be a good match with the demands of a particular situation. The ADD traits that do cause you trouble will show up quickly in the workplace. Maybe your job is simply the wrong one for you, or your employers may not know how to work with you to best utilize your skills.

No matter what the cause of the difficulty, however, you are stuck with the responsibility to make your situation workable. That's what I intend to help you with in this book: I want you to know that you have the power to be in control of yourself on the job.

Regardless of whether you are ADD or just have a few ADD traits, you need to work on whatever ADD traits you have. The goal is not so much to change them, as to realize the impact they have on you and others around you. When your awareness of those behaviors is heightened, you can decide what to do about them. You can either work on changing a trait, or you can help yourself and others learn to live with it better.

You need to learn how to accommodate your ADD wiring. This doesn't mean you or the people around you should jump through hoops. What it means is that you need to learn how to identify and meet your needs, so that you can be productive and successful in the workplace.

For example, if you are tall, you might need a chair of a different height than if you were short. If you are short, perhaps a footstool would help. If you have difficulty hearing, you might need to sit in a particular location during meetings. These are all accommodations to the differences between people.

When you consider what accommodations to make, ask yourself, "What can I contribute? And what do I need someone else to contribute?" For example, with an appliance or other machine that was new to me, I have learned to ask others to show me *how* it worked, rather than reading a lengthy instruction manual myself. That's because I know I learn best by being shown something and then practicing. That is one way I have learned to accommodate my ADD traits.

Whatever specific accommodations you need to make, the goal is to put you in control of yourself and your impact on those around you. Maximizing your potential means knowing yourself well—your stronger points and your weaker points—and learning how to make adjustments in your behavior or activities when necessary. Finding the success you deserve requires that you do what fits you best, personally and on the job. You are the one who has to take responsibility for this.

Suppose that the chair you use at work is at an inappropriate height for you and gives you leg cramps. It's okay to ask your employer to help you find a new chair, but it's ultimately your responsibility to remedy the physical discomfort caused by your chair and that is keeping you from being as productive as you could be. If worse comes to worse, maybe you even need to get out there and buy your own chair, instead of demanding that the boss do it.

In a way, the accommodations you need to make for your ADD are a lot like finding that new chair. You can moan and groan about "poor me: I have ADD, so I need . . . " But after a fairly short while, your coworkers and employers are going to get tired of this, because, let's face it, all workers have gripes and problems.

Rather than just complain, you can figure out what's bothering you and do your best to go out there and fix it. It isn't always easy, but this book will help you identify your difficulties in the workplace and suggest ways to solve them.

I hope that our workplace and educational systems learn to accommodate differences more readily. Until they do, *you* do what you can to take care of yourself. Then strive to find ways to change the systems for all people.

Different Types of ADD

If you think you might have ADD, if ADD traits seem to explain some problems you are having, you need to seek a professional diagnosis. ADD is a complex condition, not something you can diagnose yourself after reading one book or talking to some friends who have it. You need to work with a professional who is very familiar with it.

If you have already been professionally diagnosed as being ADD, that evaluation should have given you a sense of ADD's specific impact. Do you tend to have more problems with impulsivity or with being distracted? Does organization throw you into a frenzy, or is your hypersensitivity your biggest liability?

From your diagnosis or evaluation, I hope that you have learned which of the three major types of ADD you have and that you have received recommendations for dealing with your ADD traits.

During the past ten years, I have become aware of three major types of ADD. Each presents a different face of ADD. The three faces are **Outwardly Expressive ADD**, which often presents as an Active Entertainer; **Inwardly Directed ADD**, which presents as the Restless Dreamer; and **Highly Structured ADD**, which frequently presents as a Conscientious Controller.

A person with **Outwardly Expressive ADD** will appear hyperactive both verbally and physically, be impulsive and outgoing, and will tend to take on more at one time than any ten people can accomplish. This type of person loves an audience; usually has a great sense of humor; and is dramatic, expressive, and very people-friendly. People with this type of ADD gravitate to sales, high-risk occupations, and the entertainment business, often becoming entrepreneurs.

People with **Inwardly Directed ADD** are frequently craftsmen and artists, mechanically inclined or "techies," caregivers and helpers, or people who love the outdoors. Often quiet, restless, and thinking about things rather than doing things, they are also impulsive and sensitive—but you wouldn't always know that just by looking at the person.

People with **Highly Structured ADD** tend to be very controlling and hyperfocused and to require structure to function. If one piece of their structure is changed, they are likely to come unglued, rant and rave, and create chaos. Prone to blaming others, they have a tough time with relationships and negotiation. People with this type of ADD gravitate to the military and accounting, work as airline pilots or at anything requiring details and a highly structured format.

When you know which type of ADD predominates for you, you will have a better idea of what your strengths and liabilities are, what you need, and how you can accommodate those needs. Some people are primarily one or the other of the three types, and some people are a mixture of two or more types. Families often reflect a variety of types from member to member. Although we do know that ADD is genetic and passed from parent to child, we don't see any relationships yet between the type of ADD that a parent has and the type exhibited by the child.

What's important for you is to know how your ADD expresses itself through you as an individual. No one type of ADD is better or worse than any other type, just as having ADD is not better or worse than not having it. Let's remember that differences are only differences, and that each of us has his or her own assets and liabilities to work with.

The purpose of this book is to help you make adjustments for the way you are, not to change you into a non-ADD person. I want you to clearly choose what you want to modify in yourself so that you can have the best chance possible to take advantage of opportunities that come your way at work. I want you to know what you can change about yourself and when you need to go for help. I want you to learn how to ask for that help. And I want you to know how others may perceive you, so you can head off any incorrect perceptions before they hurt you or your effectiveness.

Yes, I am glad I am ADD. I want you to be glad you are ADD, too. Then you can make the contributions we all need for you to make, and you can live up to the wonderful potential you have.

Go for it!

2

Behavioral Issues That Affect Your Job

Although you can look like the most impressive job candidate to ever walk in the door—an impressive degree from a well-respected university, a grade point average that anyone would envy, and a list of community service work a mile long—none of your credentials necessarily means you're equipped to be successful in the workplace if you have ADD.

Your education might have taught you how to produce an accurate profit-and-loss statement. However, chances are no one taught you how to deal with the frustration of trying to produce that statement in the middle of a noisy, chaotic office. Or how do you deal with a boss who looks over your shoulder twenty times a day? Or how do you deal with the distraction of the secretary's radio as it announces exactly when to call in for the next contest?

"And for those of you who are listening at work . . . ," the deejay says.

Listening at work? Who are they kidding? Can anyone actually get any work done in a place like this? The answer is yes, some people can. For people with ADD, though, chances are it's going to be pretty difficult.

Let's take a look at some of the "real-world" workplace situations in which you're likely to find yourself. Let's see what effects your ADD might have on your behavior and how you can work with your ADD to be successful at your job.

We'll start with Roberto. Roberto has a degree in finance from a good university and was thrilled when he was hired by a large investment company. He understands his assignments very clearly and has every intention of giving his supervisor exactly what he asks for.

But Roberto can't seem to get anything done. His "office" consists of a small work carrel in the middle of a roomful of carrels. The sides of the carrel do not screen out any noise and are so low that he has a clear view of almost everything in the room.

Roberto is not aware that he has ADD and that he could work successfully if he would just change a few aspects of his environment. Instead, he is falling further and further behind on his assignments and living in fear that his boss will notice. Because of that fear, he becomes impatient with anyone who interrupts him to ask a question, and his temper flares with little warning. His colleagues talk and laugh as they leave the office in small groups for lunch, but Roberto asks aloud, "Doesn't anyone around here care about getting any work done?"

In an attempt to hide his lack of productivity, Roberto never asked his supervisor for a quieter place to work. Nor does he ask to come in early or stay late. His boss, not knowing what is causing Roberto's irritability and temper problems, thinks he might have an unstable employee on his hands. He begins to look for ways to let Roberto go.

Then there's Jimmy, a software developer. Jimmy knows he has ADD and knows what resources he needs to do his job well. Although he initially felt overwhelmed when the goals and demands of the day were reviewed at the daily team meetings, he has learned to sit at the back of the room and remain silent until things begin to make sense to him. Usually he gets the picture within ten minutes or so. Then he speaks up and leads the group in constructive planning for the project at hand. His teammates consider Jimmy a strong, valuable asset to the team.

Jimmy's boss, however, sees things differently. Rushing up to Jimmy with a question, he demands an instant answer. When Jimmy says he'll be back with the answer in ten minutes, the boss yells, "That's not good enough. What's wrong with you? I need an answer now, not later!"

If some of Roberto's and Jimmy's problems sound familiar to you, you may be discovering additional effects of your ADD. Many people with ADD recognize that their ADD affects their behavior in some ways, but you might not have realized the *extent* to which your ADD affects your behavior and your interaction with your peers. Common behaviors attributed to ADD include hypersensitivity, temper, impulsivity; clowning around, not appearing to take things seriously; distractibility, poor ability to focus on one issue at a time; and needing to learn by doing something rather than by just hearing or reading about it.

You might never have recognized, however, the flip side to each of these behaviors, which can work in your favor in the workplace. For example, take hypersensitivity. What hypersensitivity means to you is that you feel things acutely, and you tend to get your feelings hurt easily. When that happens, you are likely to *react* to what others do and say. You may even feel depressed or angry as the result of ordinary criticism.

That same trait of hypersensitivity, though, probably makes you good at figuring out all kinds of problems. When you are talking to others, you can figure out a lot about them by what they're saying. Also, you are sensitive to what they don't tell you; you can even pick up on things they don't necessarily want you to know about. You often can figure out the next move someone else is going to make.

Any job dependent on excellent intuition or empathy will benefit from your skills. If you are mechanically inclined, you may know intuitively what's wrong with a machine or a program. You make a good troubleshooter, inventor, or fixer. You just get into the job and make things happen.

I bet you can name a dozen instances in which your temper, impulsivity, and impatience caused you to act first without thinking. Chances are, you paid the price of reduced effectiveness on the job for that behavior. But if you have a temper, you have a high amount of energy that you can use to your advantage—if you harness it. Your impulsivity, properly managed, can become spontaneity—a positive attribute in many situations. Your impatience, properly harnessed, can help you get things done in a timely manner.

Even clowning around can be used to your advantage if you learn there is a time and a place for it. If you continuously fail to take things or people seriously, your colleagues' nerves will probably suffer. On the other hand, your good sense of humor can be used to ease a lot of tense situations. In some jobs, like customer service, a sense of humor is a great asset. In any work environment, it usually boosts morale.

Distractibility, the best-known symptom of ADD, can certainly get you off track. In a goal-oriented project, your lack of focus could raise production costs, delay completion of a job, and alienate coworkers. However, when you are called upon to be creative, the ability to think along multiple tracks at the same time is a great advantage.

Finally, many people with ADD are at a disadvantage because of the need to learn things by doing rather than by learning from someone else's experience. Such experimentation can consume time and increase costs. People who learn by doing, however, tend to retain information and strategies for use on other projects. New ways of doing things evolve when you bring your fresh approach to an old task.

Remember, although your ADD-related behaviors can cause problems in a work environment, they can also be used in a constructive way to your advantage. ADD is, after all, only a different way of being wired, and that means you do things in a unique way—not a wrong way, just a different way.

Hypersensitivity: The Problem

Cecilia waits tables and sometimes tends bar for a moderately priced, family-style restaurant. Although the pay is modest and most of the tips are low, she enjoys the laid-back attitude of the customers and feels comfortable, so she has kept the job for several years.

Cecilia begins to look at her life with a new perspective after being diagnosed with ADD, though. She thinks about the fact that she had failed every time she tried college. Unlike her sister and mom, who also have ADD, Cecilia is quiet and not able to talk her way through difficult situations. The new diagnosis of Inwardly Expressive ADD has given her new understanding of herself. She thinks that maybe she can succeed in school after all and get a better-paying job.

Cecilia interviews at an upscale restaurant with a clientele that tips well, in order to save money for tuition, and is hired. After the first day of training, she is a nervous wreck. Unlike her former employer, the management of this restaurant has very precise ways of doing things, and she fears she'll forget and get into trouble.

After she has worked three shifts, the manager questions Cecilia about a disgruntled businessman who complained about her. They discuss the situation, and the manager says, "We have high standards for our help. I'm sure you'll catch on." The restaurant is packed, and the manager is under pressure; not realizing how sensitive Cecilia is, he doesn't take the time to reassure her at length that she's really doing a very good job.

In response to what she perceives as severe criticism, Cecilia feels humiliated and mortified. She immediately quits and goes back to her old job.

Cecilia's hypersensitivity caused her to run away from making changes in her life. With her hopes for an increased income gone, she immediately gave up her plans to enroll in school. She was afraid that if she *did* go to school again, she would get something wrong anyway and not be able to please the professors. She decided she'd better play it safe and stick with what she knew.

This hypersensitivity to criticism is not uncommon with people who have ADD. When you are used to "goofing up," or not getting things right according to the way *others* define "right," you will tend to expect criticism, even imagining it when it doesn't exist. When it doesn't come from other people, you may be self-critical. In addition, you feel, see, hear, and sense things acutely, picking up small nuances of others' expressions.

Do you always assume, in all situations, that you are to blame for all problems? Conversely, do you always find fault with the person doing the criticizing, thus defending yourself against hurt?

Each and every misunderstanding or hurtful situation on a job cannot be talked through and analyzed. There isn't time for coworkers or supervisors to explain everything they say and the motive behind each of the comments. Consequently, people with ADD, and the hypersensitivity that can come with it, can spend a lot of time in the workplace with hurt feelings.

Coworkers, not always sure how to handle the situation, often say, "You're too sensitive. Don't feel that way." But that's like telling a fair-skinned person, "Don't sunburn. You shouldn't feel it."

Hypersensitivity: What You Can Do

For your own well-being, though, you have to learn to protect yourself from both real and perceived hurt from others, or you will turn work into a painful experience and the workplace into a therapeutic arena. You can begin to protect yourself by realizing that every grouchy word, grimace, or moment of silence does not necessarily have anything to do with you. The other person might have eaten something that didn't sit right in his stomach, or maybe a fight with his wife got his whole day off to a bad start. Maybe his boss just chewed him out, and you are only seeing his leftover discomfort.

Concentrate on yourself instead of your coworkers. What you believe about yourself is your best protection against being hurt, so recognize your skills and the fact that you are a valuable person. In all probability, your company did not make a mistake when it hired you (though it's common for people with ADD to think that an error must have been made). Your employer had confidence that you could do the job that was needed, and do it well. If you're self-employed, rest assured that you are probably as adequate as the next guy.

When you are around someone who is insensitive, says hurtful things, or is acting like a buffoon, say to yourself silently that you are okay. "I am fine. I will stay calm, cool, and collected." Take a deep breath and keep your attention on the facts, not the way the person talks.

People with ADD do well to learn a modest form of self-hypnosis that can be instantly put into operation when needed. Concentrate on your breathing first. Then focus your attention inward rather than on the other person, though you continue to look at him. Speak to yourself calmly with words you have trained yourself to use, such as "I'm okay."

Another option is simply to say to the outspoken person, "I'm leaving now. I will talk to you when things have calmed down." Then leave. Though some bosses may not allow you to do that, it's usually a good idea with coworkers. Even with clients, you can excuse yourself for a moment so you can count to ten and compose yourself.

When you are responsible for upsetting another person, it's important to recognize when that person is overreacting. After all, that person might be jumping to conclusions, too. Coworkers sometimes display their emotions loudly and speak before they have a chance to think. You will tend to calm them down by softening your voice and using your empathy to understand them.

With these kinds of techniques, you may not escape *feeling* hurt, but you will not feel so helpless. Then, when you are away from the situation, talk to someone who can empathize with you and nurture you.

If you are hypersensitive, you need to develop a sense of emotional power, the power to defend and protect yourself. Some people like to visualize themselves surrounded by a wall or some form of protection. I personally like to visualize having a full-length magic cloak that deflects hurtful words and actions. I visualize the cloak being thrown over my shoulders, and it has a hood I can pull up if a situation is particularly stressful.

You also have the power to walk away, quit your job, or refuse to serve someone who is abusive. You are never *permanently* trapped, even though you may need to stay in the stressful situation until you can find another job.

Remember, your hypersensitivity requires that you protect yourself. Please give yourself permission to place yourself in supportive, friendly environments. Know that you do not need to remain indefinitely in any situation that is hurtful. If someone says to you, "You're too sensitive," just say, "I am as sensitive as I am, and I intend to protect myself."

The outcome for Cecilia could have been different if she had known how to be self-supportive and talk to herself in an empowering and nurturing way. She could have said silently, "I am doing fine for the first week. Everyone makes mistakes, and I will learn. I can talk with the boss when the restaurant is less crowded, if he continues to seem irritated with me."

The Flip Side of Hypersensitivity: A Strong Sense of Intuition

Being hypersensitive is difficult and sometimes painful. But it does have a flip side that can serve as a tremendous asset for you in the workplace: a keen sense of intuition. Most of the business world's top salespeople have good intuition, often called a gut-level feeling. For example, successful salespeople seem to just *know* with whom to spend their time, when to close a deal, and what the other person needs in order to be satisfied. Believing in and depending on this sense of intuition pays rich dividends.

All healers, teachers, and counselors, and anyone working with the public, can use this positive side of hypersensitivity to great advantage. The ability to sense what is wrong with someone, even if that someone isn't aware of the problem, is a gift that ADD brings.

Probably one of my greatest strengths in my thirty years as a counselor came from this aspect of my ADD. I learned to trust my gut-level feelings. That *intuition* is always right. I do not go wrong unless I try to fight against that intuitive sense, like if I second-guess myself for the sake of logic or some empirical measurement.

A sense of timing—and this is different from telling time or being on time—is dependent upon sensitivity to others and their environment. Creative approaches to many projects and endeavors are built on the foundation of hypersensitivity in all of its ramifications.

Unfortunately, many people in academic, scientific, and midlevel management positions today do not have ADD. Because they do not have experience with this style of perceiving and finding answers, they do not tend to believe in it.

Likewise unfortunately, over the last few years the mental health and medical fields have shifted from emphasizing the hands-on healer who knows his trade to valuing expensive testing and reams of paperwork to justify results that frequently could be unearthed with sensitivity. Even the diagnosis and treatment of ADD has succumbed to overtesting to "prove" empirically that someone has ADD. Professionals need to be allowed to draw from their strengths, whether that means taking an intuitive or an empirical approach. Professionals who have ADD would be especially strengthened by developing their intuition and using it to help their patients or clients.

Temper, Impulsivity, and Impatience: The Problem

Frank, a big, hulking man, got in trouble on his job as a warehouseman. Although he is smart, strong, and reliable, his temper and impulsivity keep him from getting ahead. Frank always has said whatever he thinks, not stopping to consider the consequences. When he became mad one day because a substitute supervisor blamed him for a foul-up—one for which he wasn't responsible—he glared at the man, wheeled around, and muttered, "Damn, f____' b____!" Frank walked off the job ten minutes before the lunch whistle blew.

When he returned on time from lunch, Frank had cooled off and pretty much forgotten the incident. His boss hadn't, though, and wanted to talk about what had happened. Fearful of being criticized, Frank immediately got "hot" again and refused to listen to what the man had to say. He forgot that his rent was due, that his kids needed new clothes for school, and that his wife needed to get some expensive dental work done.

"You can take this job!" Frank yelled at his boss. "I quit."

Frank was extremely sensitive, and he felt enormous emotional pain when anything about his character or work was questioned. He took pride in being responsible, and anyone who worked around him for even a short while knew it. Unfortunately, though, this wasn't the first time Frank had quit a job impulsively, without first laying plans for getting another one.

Never having graduated from high school, Frank developed the habit of working extra hard to make up for his lack of education. Unable to sit still in school or pay attention to bookwork, he had felt frustrated trying to do assignments. He could understand what the teachers were saying, but he simply couldn't concentrate long enough to complete worksheets or papers or take tests satisfactorily.

By junior high Frank felt so stressed by the gap between how smart he was and his ability to produce in school that he wanted to quit. A coach talked him into playing ball because of his size. He played well, and he could memorize the plays when the coach showed him what he wanted. But when he flunked two subjects after the first six weeks of school and was grounded from playing, he walked out of school and never returned.

Leaving school was a very painful experience for Frank. He couldn't even bear to think about it. He had tried as hard as he could to understand the coursework, but his mind wouldn't work right, and no one seemed to understand that. No one would listen to him, so he stopped trying to tell anyone what was happening.

Now, years later, he was in the habit of simply blowing up and walking away from situation after situation. What was the use of trying?

With ADD, temper explosions and impulsive behavior are commonplace due to an inability to delay action until thinking about a situation, coupled with a flood of hurt feelings from hypersensitivity. Angry feelings are likely to result as a defense against feeling helpless, fearful, and frustrated. When that anger is not channeled constructively, it scatters out like shotgun pellets in the form of temper outbursts.

When a person is in severe emotional pain, immediate action, such as a temper tantrum, carries him away from the source of the pain. The person's immediate goal at that time is to protect himself. He isn't really thinking about what the results of that behavior will be.

If you have ADD and are prone to outbursts of temper, what you must realize is that great sensitivity underlies your outbursts. You are lashing out against others in an attempt to protect yourself against the depth of your feelings.

Understanding that is only one step in the right direction. Your next step is to retrain yourself so you will have alternative ways to protect yourself without lashing out at other people.

Having learned that you may forget or fail to follow through on things, you are likely to become very fidgety when you have to wait—and that includes while waiting instead of lashing out immediately upon feeling hurt. The discomfort that comes from trying to remain still, as well as the concern that you'll forget to do or say something that's important to you, leads to feelings of impatience. Fear that you will not reach a goal creates a sense of powerlessness. Better do it right away, your fear says, and your impulsive behavior begins.

You have developed that impatience in order to protect yourself. The truth is, however, that others usually don't see it that way. They are likely to view you as pushy, poorly disciplined, or selfish. Unless they also have ADD, they probably don't understand what it feels like to live inside your body. But you know: the buildup of pressure is enormous, and action, or at least a plan of action, is the only thing that helps you feel better.

The whole trick is to figure out ways to tolerate reasonable amounts of inaction without losing track of your goals and well-being.

Temper, Impulsivity, and Impatience: What You Can Do

Temper, impulsivity, and impatience can be managed if you are willing to take several steps.

First, you must commit to work on each condition. Don't agree to do that because someone else says you should. Commit to working on this issue only if you really want to find alternative ways to deal with your feelings and get what you want.

Next, you must be willing to make some changes in your work life. Sometimes it's even necessary to change where you work or the kind of work you are doing, if you're in a work environment that just doesn't suit you. Blowing up at colleagues, impulsively buying new things, or impatiently snapping at employees who are trying to learn their jobs are all indicators that you may be in an environment that just isn't right for you. If city life stresses you, a small-town environment may suit you much better.

This doesn't mean you have to walk off your job tomorrow, but it does mean that you need to begin to plan for future changes. Think about how you would really like to live. Inventory your skills. Most importantly, listen to your heart and begin to trust your feelings. Watch for opportunities, no matter how different from what you have been doing, that would free you to live in the manner you would like. The changes will come to pass if you are willing to allow them.

You must next learn the cues that trigger your temper, impulsivity, and impatience. To recognize these cues, here's what you have to do:

1. Think of the last time your temper flared or you acted out of impatience or impulsivity.

2. Ask yourself what you were doing right beforehand. You will begin to see typical problems that set you up or trigger your temper, impulsivity, or impatience.

3. Go to the person you interacted with and apologize for losing your temper or acting impulsively or impatiently.

4. Congratulate yourself on beginning to stop the process of being ruled by these ineffective behaviors.

5. Ask the person to help you the next time you seem to be getting out of control. Agree on a signal, for example the time-out signal used by referees in sporting events. Agree that when either of you makes the sign, you immediately back off and give yourself a chance to come up with alternative ways to get what you need, short-circuiting your automatic behavior. This form of a buddy system can work exceedingly well on the job.

6. Every new time you feel the pressure of temper, impulsivity, or impatience, do the same things listed in steps 2 through 5. You will find that it takes you less time to remedy the situation each time you go through the process. Eventually, you will catch yourself before you act.

7. Remember to keep a sharp lookout for situations that tend to make you angry or stressed.

The Flip Side of Temper, Impulsivity, and Impatience

Lashing out at someone in a rage of temper takes a lot of energy, so we know that anyone whose temper flares out of control has a lot of energy at his or her disposal. Channeled properly, it can be utilized to drive a powerful, goal-oriented "attack" on an issue or situation.

For example, if you are unjustly fired from a job, you may choose to lash out at your boss. On the other hand, using the energy from your anger, you can choose to set up a competing company. You might just end up beating the competition.

If you are impulsive, that means you can do things quickly. With training, that quickness can help you respond in the blink of an eye to a situation that takes others longer to identify. Many a star football running back, with the intuitive ability to "find the hole," is actually responding impulsively to situations that become available for a very short period of time.

Great business deals have been made quickly by someone with educated impulsivity. Knowing your business allows you to respond immediately to opportunity when it presents itself.

Being impatient is a good quality if you become impatient with situations that really are offensive. Then your impatience can be a positive force for stopping them. For example, impatience with abuse, neglect, or anything hurtful to people leads to needed action. Positive change at all levels of our society can occur when someone gets impatient with the status quo. However, the trick is to be clear about what you're impatient about and why you are impatient—and what your goal should be when you take action.

Your job as someone with ADD is to gain control over your behaviors so that you can make them assets. You may find you need to explain to someone who is wired differently what it feels like inside you. If the expression of your emotions and your behavior are under *your* control, you will find that many non-ADD people will listen to you and begin to understand what life is like for those who are different.

Speak up, then take a look at how the two of you can work as a team.

Clowning Around

Coworkers called Janice the funniest person they'd ever met. She was always clowning around the shop, dropping one-liners as deftly as others breathe. She was at her most raucous at the end of the month, when the crunch was on and projects needed to be completed. When a customer walked in, she'd often slyly mimic the person. Sometimes she wasn't very subtle, but she figured people ought to be able to take a little kidding. The office staff and shop personnel had been together for a long time, and everyone was so used to Janice's behavior that no one talked about it.

It was only after a new person, Allison, was hired that Janice's clowning around began to be seen as a problem. Allison felt irritated by Janice's horseplay. At first, Allison thought her nerves were edgy because of all she had to learn. She found herself staying late quite often, but assumed that was because she hadn't completely learned her new job yet. Then she began to notice that she was doing much more than half the work she and Janice were supposed to share. She realized that Janice handled only the accounts that were straightforward and gave Allison the difficult accounts to straighten out.

When Allison mentioned the situation to other people in her department, they told her not to be so serious. Soon these same workers began to come to Allison to share that Janice's kidding around sometimes caused troubles for them, also.

The truth was that Janice, like many people with ADD, felt chronically inadequate at her job, but she never mentioned these feelings to anyone. Instead, she joked and teased, distracting attention away from the real issues.

Many people with ADD are naturally quick-witted. They rapidly make unusual connections between events. When those connections are verbalized, they are often very funny. And that's fine. What's not so fine is when the humor is used to distract others, and the humorist, too, from real issues at hand.

Sometimes humor is a vehicle to convey anger toward others. You will recognize this type of humor as put-downs, making fun of others, or prejudicial humor. It is never funny!

What to Do about Negative Clowning Behavior

Healthy clowning behavior livens up any work situation, especially if the humor is not abusive. But when it overreaches acceptable standards, is used to cover up deficiencies, or interferes with business, it's time to do something about it.

The first step is to become aware of the humor and assess its effects. Whether you are looking at your own use of humor or another's, think back about when the clowning around occurs, what is going on, and what is said or done.

Next you must determine the function that the humor is playing. Is it a cover-up for feelings of inadequacy, anxiety, or emotional pain? Does it communicate anger or prejudice? More than one of these may underlie someone's clowning.

If you're dealing with another person, go to that person in a quiet moment in private. Tell him or her that sometimes you appreciate humor, but sometimes it bothers you. If you are a supervisor or other boss to the person, you can say it is causing a problem in the workplace. Also say you are concerned about the person and suspect there are some very sensitive feelings under the humor. Speak directly, offer to listen, but also tell the person it is okay if he or she prefers not to share. The message is that you are willing to help out, but the inappropriate use of humor must stop.

If you are a supervisor, be sure to let the person know you appreciate any improvement. Remember, people with ADD are very sensitive. However, do be firm and watch out that you don't get caught back up in the horseplay. It's very infectious.

The Flip Side of Clowning Around

Many a work setting has benefited from seeing the light side of situations. Laughing about those things in life that we can do nothing about tends to relieve the harshness of the feelings of helplessness. Humor keeps people from burning out when stress gets too intense.

Some guidelines are needed, however. Laughing about ourselves is fine; laughing about another person is not. Using humor in balance with seriousness, as called for by the situation, can be an asset. Using humor to experience the joys of life is fine. Humor as a cover-up for feelings is not. Repeatedly faking your way through situations by clowning around is not.

When you have done all you can to figure out what to do about your ADD, there may come good times to step in with humor.

For example, I cannot tell you how conscientiously I have tried to keep track of expenses, time charts, and mileage. No matter how hard I work at it, I simply forget to pay attention to the details of all those little numbers. Finally, I have come to the place where I simply laugh. Facetiously, I might say to my secretary, "Here, give me the office receipts. I'll draw up the financial statement." She and I always get a good laugh out of that—and I promise you, she actually becomes eager to tally the records. She knows that's a lot better than trying to unscramble the mess I would make.

Distractibility

Have you ever found yourself in a situation where your boss is telling you about a new assignment that is interesting to you, is very important to the company, and demonstrates your boss's confidence in you, only to discover partway into his presentation that your thoughts are on a completely different subject? For people with ADD, this is a common occurrence.

Gerald, a top salesman for his company, has earned a prestigious assignment: introducing a new line of products to a new territory. The job includes training sales staff, which he loves to do, and serving as the key representative for his company. He feels very good about his boss's confidence in him. Yet, while his boss is discussing the assignment with him, he suddenly realizes that he's completely tuned out to the details his boss is giving him. He prays his boss will repeat the information.

Where did Gerald go mentally? Well, first, he noticed the picture on his boss's desk, the one taken during last winter's vacation in Colorado. He wondered if his new sales territory includes Colorado. If it does, will he be able to establish an office that is within easy driving distance of the ski slopes? He recalled how much he enjoys skiing. The next thing he knew, he'd mentally designed a whole presentation to his boss about where the office should be and why. Meanwhile, he never heard the boss tell him that Colorado is a part of the plan and he can choose any location he wants for the office.

The worst part about the distractibility associated with ADD is that there is no warning that it is about to happen. You only know afterwards—when you have no idea what you've missed—that you weren't paying attention. It has little to do with whether you *intend* to pay attention, and that is extremely hard to understand for people who are not distractible.

If you have ADD, the distractions can come from within your mind. That is, you find yourself thinking about several things at once or sequentially moving from one thought to another. However, there is always a logic behind the direction your thoughts take; they *are* connected. The problem is that they usually move away from the task at hand.

You may be bothered by what you see, hear, smell, taste, or feel. The rough upholstery pressing against the back of your leg catches your attention. Smells drift from the microwave popcorn in an adjoining room, or you become aware of the residual taste of onions from lunch. Each of these produces a potential pathway for your thoughts to drift away from the topic at hand.

You may also be distracted by picking up the feelings of others. When someone enters your office angry, even though the person might be smiling, you probably experience the anger. When a coworker is anxious about holding up his end of the deal, you probably empathize with it and may even get nervous in return, becoming distracted. Perhaps you realize that it is only the other person who is having the trouble, but you begin to think about him or her and what may be causing the trouble. Off your mind goes again.

What You Can Do about Distractibility

First and foremost, you must find a way to deal with this that fits you— one you can use time and time again, automatically. Because the way you tune out sound is automatic, you must intervene in the same way to save yourself. The following are only suggestions; try any that feel plausible to you. If one works, use it. Otherwise, try another tactic.

Keeping my hands busy helps me maintain attention to others. I like to do some form of handwork best; knitting or bead stringing is great in big meetings. The repetitive nature of the task suits me well because my thinking mind can focus on what is being said. If I get caught without handiwork, though, I might pick up a pen and draw or doodle. That is a more creative process, however, and more easily takes my attention away from the speaker.

Interestingly, writing has become much easier for me now that word processors have replaced handwriting. In the past I always became sleepy as soon as I sat down to write. Typewriters didn't work for me, either, because my train of thought kept getting broken by changing paper, shifting lines, and correcting errors. Now the physical activity of typing at the processor helps me pay attention, and I can work for long periods of time without a break.

Taking notes on what is being said works well when I am meeting with someone directly. I have also found that remaining standing helps me focus my attention, especially if I move around the room while having a discussion. You might find that taping what is being said for later review works. One insurance salesman I know immediately dictates notes about what he is going to do about what he has been hearing.

If you are aware that you missed a point, do not hesitate to ask someone to repeat or clarify what was said. That way, you will have the information you need, and the process of asking for clarification will help you focus your attention better next time. This is not an excuse to be sloppy. Try the best you can to keep on track; otherwise, you are being rude to the person talking. But sometimes what is being said triggers so many wonderful thoughts that it's a compliment to tell the person so, then ask for a repetition of what was said.

Highlighting written material can help you focus. I like to make notes in the columns of books about what I'm reading, either in outline form or in response to the author. Sometimes I focus better when I read aloud. Despite popularly held beliefs to the contrary, leaving a radio, television, or fan on assists some people with ADD to pay attention when they are working. Others report they must have absolute silence to work, sometimes doing much better starting work when others have gone to bed. For these reasons, flex time, where the exact hours of work are left up to the individual, is great for people with ADD.

For some people with ADD, medication helps concentration. Certainly for anyone who has a lot of work that is hard to focus on and where attention lapses cause great trouble, the proper prescription of medication can be indicated. Students and those whose jobs sporadically require intense concentration may benefit from medication at those times. Consult with your physician about types and usage of medication.

Ironically, some of the most intense situations do not require outside help. Emergency and crisis work, and any high-intensity work, creates an excellent focus on the task at hand.

The bigger problems usually come with repetitive, mundane, boring tasks that do not stimulate someone with ADD enough to keep their attention. You may wish to break these tasks into small segments, rewarding yourself with breaks that reinforce your productivity. For example, thirty concentrated minutes of paying bills may deserve a reward of walking around the block or watching a little TV. Your job is to set a limit on the reward so you return to the task in a timely manner.

The Flip Side of Distractibility: Multiple-Track Awareness

Though I didn't know I had ADD when I was a radio talk show host, I discovered a talent that was the result of my ADD: I could think and talk on five levels at once when a caller asked a question.

First, I heard the specific question being asked. Simultaneously, I thought about what the motivation of the person might be or what lay behind the question. I was also aware of the needs of the other listeners and the station manager's desires about programming. Finally, I kept track of the mechanics of the show, such as time spent on the line with the caller, proximity to break time, and special communications from my producer and technical director. All five levels operated simultaneously in my head while I was listening and talking. I enjoyed it immensely, and nothing could distract me from my job because that job itself involved so much stimulation.

Finding patterns in what is going on around you at work is another ADD talent. For example, you might be involved with one agenda, such as selling a product, while at the same time be aware that this sale may be a lead for another product. Much networking between people involves seeing a situation's potential to spin off further situations to follow up on. All creative, inventive collaborations are influenced by multitrack processing of information.

Heightened awareness is excellent if you are working in a situation that is potentially dangerous. An extreme example of this is experienced by soldiers who serve as point men, leading their troops safely into enemy territory. On a more moderate level, factory workers benefit from those who can be aware that everything all around them is progressing smoothly and safely. Airline pilots must constantly scan their instruments and note changes in the environment that could effect the plane's safety. Finally, all the troubleshooters of the world—whether mechanical, psychological, or financial—benefit from being able see many things at once and recognize various combinations of information that can create a problem. Indeed, there is a positive side to not having unilateral concentration.

Experiential Learning

When Eric was given his own project unit at a major computer company, he was ecstatic. A computer whiz who was full of ideas, he felt he would make a lot of money for the company. One of the first tasks he outlined in his mind required him to get a grasp of some new technology that only recently had become available. He was excited about the wonderful difference it would make for his company. He knew he'd be able to learn how to use it, so he wrote a proposal to his boss that included his attendance at a training seminar on the new material. With his boss's approval, he signed up for the week-long course.

To Eric's dismay, the class was a fourteen-week course that had been condensed into one week—with no time for students to get hands-on computer experience between classes. By the second day, Eric knew he was in trouble. He understood what the professor was saying at the time he was saying it, but to really learn it, he had to apply it; otherwise, he forgot what was being taught. Eric became overwhelmed, then discouraged, and finally walked out before the end of the course. What could he tell his boss?

If you have ADD, the odds are good that you will learn best with a hands-on approach. Though the process is slower, what you learn tends to stick. This is especially true when trying to learn things that are detailed, have a number of sequential steps, or are abstract.

Though ADD is not related to intelligence, people with Outwardly Expressive and Inwardly Directed ADD appear to learn more slowly due to the way in which they acquired learning. Most education is designed for people who are different from those who have these kinds of ADD. The one exception is the person who overfocuses because of having Highly Structured ADD. If you have this type of ADD, you probably like definite order to your learning enterprises and become frustrated when it is missing.

If you are the type of person who can get into a situation and feel your way through, creating new or innovative ways of handling things on the spot, you have "street smarts." This means you learn experientially, another advantage that comes from being ADD.

Dealing with Experiential Learning

If you are an experiential learner, the most important thing you can do is to speak up and let those teaching you know how you learn. Others cannot read your mind and, frankly, few people know that there are different styles of learning, so it becomes your responsibility to teach them. Use the words "show me." Tell the person that it may take a few trials for you to get the knack of something, but that once you've learned it, you're extremely reliable and loyal, and you will do a good job.

Consider Sylvia, an office worker who is put in charge of the copy machine. It is not realistic to give her a manual and expect her to be able to fix the machine if it gets jammed. Though she'll try and try, she won't understand what she's read well enough to apply it effectively to her job. Even if she manages to do the job one time, she might not remember what to do the next time, and she'll need to start over again.

However, show Sylvia step by step, let her practice each step until she has it down pat, and she won't forget what she's learned. She'll be able to see how each piece or step fits together with every other step. She may even end up improving on the current system.

The Flip Side of Being an Experiential Learner

When people have learned through doing, have learned experientially, chances are that information or those skills are going to be there for them the next time they are needed. In addition, the ability to respond quickly, with little or no preparation, to any situation is an asset of being an experiential learner.

You create alternative solutions to problems and find new ways to improve the way things are done. Pathfinders always work in this way. When situations change or a need arises for alternative solutions or new thinking, the experiential learner becomes a valuable commodity. In the modern world, where knowledge gained today is likely to be quickly outdated, the need for flexibility and innovation increases. Able to function by the seat of your pants, you fit well into today's world.

Different Types of ADD and Different Types of Behavior

Your behavior is very much influenced by the type or types of ADD you have. Regardless of how you were raised, certain aspects of your behavior will have been defined by your neurochemistry. Of course, your parents' wiring will reflect the way in which they raised you. Nevertheless, your own physical hardware will take precedence and guide the ways you react to everything you are exposed to. Let's look at each of the three types of ADD we discussed earlier and see how each influences behavior. If you are one type or a combination of two or all three types, you will see reflections of yourself in certain descriptions.

Outwardly Expressive ADD: The Active Entertainer

If you have Outwardly Expressive ADD, you are outgoing, active, and expressive. You act out your feelings. Your desires, hopes, and dreams are expressed openly. Almost everything about those with Outwardly Expressive ADD is obvious to other people. If you have a lot of this type of ADD, you will be in motion much of the time. Bouncing off the walls at work, running circles around everyone else, or tapping your fingers and jiggling your feet—or finding that same foot in your mouth at inopportune moments—earns you the label Outwardly Expressive.

On the go until the day is done, you may stop only to fall asleep or become a couch potato in front of the TV. It is as if you are unable to take a moderate course. At any given moment, you give life all or nothing. Powerful and easily seen, your energy may burst out as a temper tantrum. Impulsively doing something, anything, you definitely don't hide your actions. Even your clowning around may take gigantic proportions, so much so that you may entertain professionally or as an amateur.

Though your sensitivity is every bit as great as anyone else's, the way you display it may be by pretending not to care—or by caring dramatically, by suffering and complaining loudly.

As an outwardly expressive person, you must learn to harness your impulsivity on the job so that you don't get yourself or the company into trouble. No more fighting with a competitor. No more writing a deal before you've checked your calendar and the boss's to be sure that time is available to fulfill the obligation.

You need to know how much structure you need in order to be satisfactorily efficient yet not feel trapped. You need to introduce enough change into your work mix to avoid boredom, yet without having so much that you can't keep track of things. The whole trick is to find a balance, use your assets to your advantage, and gain some control over the parts of your behavior that get you in trouble.

Professionally, you fit well into jobs that use your skills in sales and entertainment. Anything that is new and exciting draws your attention. Entrepreneurial by nature, you are not likely to fear taking risks that others would shirk from. Your high energy serves you well, as your charismatic, expressive nature lets the world know that, in fact, you have arrived.

Your type of ADD gives rise to as many good traits as problematic ones. Your job is to learn to manage what is less constructive in your behavior and showcase the positives. Once you do that, you cannot help but be a winner.

Inwardly Directed ADD: The Restless Dreamer

ADD has more than one face. Though at first glance this type of ADD is often overlooked, and therefore often goes undiagnosed, it just as frequently causes problems. If you're called a dreamer, "out to lunch," or "spacy," you may have discovered that the reason is ADD.

Inwardly directed, your behaviors are more subtly displayed than those of your Outwardly Directed counterparts. Instead of shouting angrily when someone cuts in front of you on the freeway, you may think about it, mumbling four-letter words to yourself. Coworkers may wonder why you're so irritable, snapping at anyone who gets in your way.

Though not hyperactive, you probably suffer from restlessness, finding it difficult to stay seated. You probably like being outdoors or working on something that allows you to stand and walk around. You jump to conclusions in your mind, or you fear that you'll forget what you want to say if you don't immediately jump into a conversation—such problems plague people with Inwardly Expressive ADD. Your impulsivity may come out in the form of buying things for your business without having a plan for their use. Though you probably dislike structure, your daydreaming may carry you away from goals, especially if they're not *your* goals. Your acute sensitivity coupled with a tendency to not speak up can lead to pouting, depression, and withdrawal—none of which has any place on the job.

To gain control of this form of ADD, you must be sure to listen to your heart and note how you feel. Then place yourself in situations that need the wonderful skills you have. Frequently talented, creative, and inventive, you and your companions with Inwardly Expressive ADD make the world a better place to live.

Believe in yourself and your feelings. Often you will find you are a good listener, helper, and friend. Though I'm not asking you to go completely against your grain, I do ask that you let the rest of us see what you're made of. You are valuable.

Restless Dreamers tend to gravitate to careers in the creative arts and crafts. Inventors, hands-on artisans and builders, mechanics, and "techies" of the modern computer are using ADD to an advantage. The counselors, teachers, and caregivers of the world make good use of the empathy and sensitivity inherent in this form of ADD. With selling based on loyalty and long-term relationships, the insurance industry and some other financial businesses attract people with these characteristics. Steady, agreeable, and sensitive, you find the workplace benefits from your ADD attributes.

The biggest difficulties for you to watch out for usually involve paperwork and details. Otherwise, having your own business may suit you fine.

The world needs your talents. Share and enjoy the fruits of turning what's often thought of as a liability into an asset.

Highly Structured ADD: The Conscientious Controller

Methodical, perfectionistic, and extremely conscientious, Highly Structured ADD traits may hardly seem like ADD at all. With an overdependence on structure and control, however, you suffer from distractibility and organizational problems just as much as people with the other types of ADD.

Hypersensitivity, often covered by gruffness, is pushed away so that feelings don't hurt so bad. Impulsivity and impatience take the form of a right; those not accommodating you are seen as wrong. Sometimes you cease all activity so you don't lose control.

If you have Highly Structured ADD, you may hyperfocus, sitting in one place for long periods of time, mesmerized. Unable to take no for an answer, you may pressure others against their will in an attempt to get your world ordered in such a way as to make you feel secure. Resisting change of personnel or programs, you may compulsively plan every move or action on your job. Finally, when thwarted, you have a tendency to preach at others as if they were wrong and you were right.

In the workplace, you can harness your traits, soften their edges, and become a dynamic leader. Often found at your best in highly structured settings, it would not be surprising to find you drawn toward jobs in the military, accounting, and organizational management. Airline pilots take advantage of this form of ADD, as do medical doctors, research scientists, and university professors with ADD. Clerical work benefits from the same traits. Top-notch executives and legal secretaries require the positive attributes brought by this type of ADD.

With your traits under control, remembering that other people often are not like you and cannot live up to your standards, you can be a dynamic leader, business owner, or the very glue that holds a business together. Work with others who may have more access to expressing their sensitivity. Together, with mutual respect, you can develop a dynamic team. Just don't judge your teammates.

ADD and Addictive Behaviors

One of the toughest issues for people with ADD to deal with is the relationship between ADD and addiction. Besides drugs, alcohol, and tobacco, we must also recognize other lesser-known addictions, including sex, gambling, and spending. Even food, including chocolate or vitamins, can be used in an addictive manner.

To avoid confusion, I'd like to present the idea that anything—both substances and behaviors—can be used addictively. That's because addiction covers the way in which a substance or behavior is used. If it functions in your life in some way other than its inherent intent would indicate, it may be classed as an addiction. If you are unable to stop a behavior because you are using it to distract yourself from some feeling or need, you may be facing a problem with addiction.

Obviously, this definition goes way beyond alcohol and other substance abuse. However, let's look at these first. Biochemically, some drugs are so addictive that almost anyone using them risks addiction with very little ingestion. Street drugs such as heroin and crack cocaine typically come to mind. Many people, especially young people, experiment with a wide range of street drugs—marijuana, amphetamines, and designer drugs (drugs such as ecstasy, manufactured in laboratories)— and only some people become dependent upon them physiologically. What we know now is that certain people have brain receptors that predispose them to become addicted, and others don't. Similarly, many people drink alcohol, but only some become alcohol-dependent.

Less well known, though highly addictive and even deadly, are inhalants: glue, paint products, and anything else people can sniff to get a high. These products tend to be so toxic that severe brain damage results from moderate usage.

In addition to the biochemically addictive qualities of these substances, psychological addiction also takes place if the chemical is used to escape problems, soothe emotional or physical hurts, empower you, free you, or in any way alter how you feel.

Any behavior used in this way would be labeled addictive. For example, sex is a normal part of emotionally healthy people's lives. However, if it is used to get a high or make you feel less depressed or more powerful, rather than as a loving expression toward someone special, then the behavior would be labeled addictive. Wanting or needing that high can cause you to throw caution to the wind, with desire overriding good sense. Given the dangers of unprotected sex, that high can prove deadly.

Gambling that provides the gambler's high functions in the same way: as a cover-up for pain. Then there's the exercise junkie, who must exercise or experience withdrawal symptoms of agitation, sleeplessness, irritability, and restlessness. I always remember the man who told me he became addicted to throwing clay pots at the potter's wheel. His face taking on a wistful, even blissful expression as he spoke, he noted that once he started, he couldn't stop. With his marriage in jeopardy because of the long hours he'd been spending bent over the wheel, he was faced with having to stop altogether or lose his wife.

You can also be addicted to religion. If you frantically and obsessively go to church or worship constantly to *escape* feeling inner pain or fear rather than be freed from it, you may be addicted to religion. Obviously, a sincerely spiritual or religious person seeking a balance in life is not necessarily addicted, but check the tone of your behavior and see how you're using religion.

It is easy to become addicted to violence, emergency situations, and risk taking, not to mention video games, television, and computers. Even going for counseling can become an addiction if it's not properly handled. It's all in the function that the substance or behavior serves.

The Relationship between Addictive Behaviors and ADD

Those of us professionally involved with ADD are becoming increasingly aware of the high incidence of addiction in the lives of people who have ADD. Two quite different pictures are emerging as the relationship between ADD and addiction is researched.

First, if we look at the neuroscientific research, we discover that the same brain receptors are involved in alcohol dependence and ADD. That leads to the probability of a dual diagnosis for many people: ADD and alcoholism. Besides biochemical dependence, you can have an addictive dependence on a substance or a behavior *and* have ADD. That, too, is considered a dual diagnosis, and both conditions must be treated.

Though the research is far from complete, many addictive practices, whether chemically or behaviorally based, result in a high. This high creates the specific change in your chemistry that is required to focus attention and help you become more effective and productive. That's why it's not uncommon to hear people with ADD say, "I think more clearly if I've been running" or "When I buy something new, I get excited. Then my mind becomes clear and I feel euphoric and powerful." Who wouldn't want to return to this feeling?

The second picture of ADD and addictions looks quite different. Here, the substances or behaviors are being used to self-medicate against the pain of having ADD. As soon as the ADD is appropriately diagnosed and treated, the use of the substance or behavior in question disappears or is easily managed.

When I first saw this take place, I could hardly believe my eyes. However, since then I have seen hundreds of situations in which someone's ADD was treated, and that person immediately stopped drinking too much, quit using drugs, or gave up an addictive behavior that previously had been causing problems. But it is critical to differentiate between an addiction and self-medication.

Workaholism is an addiction that can be related to ADD. An individual may work to avoid facing inner feelings of inadequacy. Of course, work can also be used as an excuse to stay away from a situation at home that feels bad, such as a marriage that long ago lost its zest.

Many people with ADD who appear to be workaholics, however, actually are not. Instead, they are working long, hard hours just to keep up in the workplace. Due to poor organizational skills and difficulty in keeping on task, it can take a person with ADD a whole lot more time to accomplish a task than someone who is better organized. In this case, work is not an addiction, though it can certainly cause similar trouble at home or in one's personal life.

Addictive Behaviors: What You Can Do

The first thing you need to do about addictive behaviors is to have a thorough evaluation by someone familiar both with addictions and with ADD. That professional must determine the way in which the substances or behaviors are being used. If a dual diagnosis is uncovered—ADD and an addictive behavior—then each problem must be treated.

Anyone facing treatment for addictions must be ready to commit unequivocally to recovery. Abstinence from, or control over the use of, the substance or behavior is a *must,* or no other treatment has any hope of succeeding. Otherwise, everyone—clinicians, the person addicted, friends, and family—are only fooling themselves.

Once the person has committed to and begun addiction treatment, simultaneous treatment for ADD is indicated and can help with the process of addiction recovery. If you have an addiction and ADD but you do not treat the ADD, then you are setting yourself up for a harder battle than is necessary. There are always some elements of your individual pain that can be directly attributable to ADD and must be addressed. However, ADD treatment and training must only proceed while you are "working your program."

In the case of an addiction that serves to self-medicate against the pain of ADD, it is wise to immediately start treatment and training for ADD. Furthermore, the addictive behavior needs to cease immediately. What you will notice is that it becomes easier to abstain from the addictive behavior if, in fact, you are dealing with self-medication. Cravings and desires seems to be readily controlled. Should a lapse in addiction control occur, an immediate reevaluation of the situation must be made, with adjustments to your program.

Sadly, many addiction-treatment programs fail to recognize the presence and impact of a person's ADD. In time, clinicians who work with addictions will understand more about ADD. Meanwhile, all of us who do understand ADD must take responsibility to educate those who have not had the opportunity to learn.

One reason it is imperative to recognize the presence of ADD is that the way people with ADD learn is different from that of others. Consequently, some of the recovery tactics that have traditionally worked well with addicts do not work well with people who have ADD. Many of the failures in addiction treatment may be due to the lack of recognition of ADD as a core issue in substance abuse.

Another reason to be aware of the presence of ADD stems from the factor of hypersensitivity. Forceful, confrontational interventions and techniques used as part of a treatment program—techniques that might work well with many people—can be experienced as abuse by people with ADD. I have seen many instances of this that required trauma-reduction techniques to overcome. That doesn't mean that firm limits and requirements should not be part of a recovery program for addicts who have ADD. It does mean that the treatment methods need to be updated to reflect what's been learned about ADD.

ADD, Addictions, and the Workplace

Probably the most important addiction issue for the workplace—and the workplace *has* become more sensitive to addiction treatment—is that many more skilled workers can be salvaged when ADD is factored in.

Catching the signs of ADD early and making work adjustments that raise productivity while lowering the incidence of addiction-related conditions—these actions create a winning situation for everyone. Sensitivity to finding a good match between each worker and his or her job not only lowers the incidence of addiction as self-medication, but leads to finding jewels in the work pool. Company-promoted training programs that identify ADD-like behaviors and train employees and supervisors to manage them go hand in hand with training for drug and alcohol abuse.

3

Getting Organized on the Job

Getting places on time, figuring out how much you can do in an hour or a day, organizing your physical workspace, and keeping track of time, tools, and information are crucial skills for job survival—but are often frustrating for people with ADD and their coworkers. In this chapter we'll discuss some solutions to these issues so that you can have a less stressful and more productive workday. We'll discuss meeting job requirements by knowing how and when to ask for help and how to use your talents efficiently, because no matter how intelligent, creative, and talented you are, a lack of organization at your workplace can cheat you of the potential to enjoy the successes you deserve.

If you, like many people with ADD, have trouble with organization, every part of your life is affected. That lack of organization has undoubtedly exposed you to much criticism over the years, even though, at least initially, you intended to conform to the system. Though often accused of being lazy or irresponsible, in reality you may have long since just given up any hope of being able to keep on top of the organizational demands of your job. No wonder you procrastinate. You weren't avoiding your work: you just didn't know how to manage the time, information, or projects facing you.

Forgive yourself for past inadequacies and learn what to do now.

The Organization of Time

Right now, you're reading this book. How much time have you set aside for reading? What will you be doing immediately after this, and at what time do you need to start that activity? Is there something you need to do right now instead of reading? If you keep reading beyond the time you have set aside, what will the impact be on the activity you are anticipating doing next?

If you're like most people with ADD, you don't usually ask yourself these kinds of questions. Instead, you probably get caught up in an activity that interests you and just keep going. What you're doing at the present time is all you're likely to be aware of. The implications for later probably don't come to your mind—much less a plan to move on to whatever is next. You stop your activity only when you are distracted, lose interest, or become bored.

Of course, experience has probably taught you that the results of not planning ahead can be disastrous, like the time you didn't complete the paperwork you brought home to finish over the weekend. Another time, maybe you failed to call ahead to let your family know you were running very late at work, forgetting that tonight was the night you'd agreed to help your spouse clean house in preparation for a dinner for your boss tomorrow.

Anger, resentment, and criticism are a few of the responses you are likely to confront when coworkers or family members become irritated about your poor sense of time. Coworkers and buddies may wash their hands of you, fearful that they'll get left holding the bag once again. You could end up wondering why. You know you're a nice person who doesn't mean to hurt anyone. Nevertheless, your failure to be on time or finish a job in a timely manner alienates people, and you don't need this.

Feeling guilty because you once again got sidetracked can spoil a good day and cheat you of using your potential. When you spend a lot of time apologizing, you use up vital energy that could be more constructively applied to your job. Also, the constant stress that comes from always being out of sync with those around you lowers your quality of life.

Different Ways of Perceiving Time

What causes trouble for people with ADD is the division of time into segments, arbitrary segments at that. If you are focused on the conversation you are having, the most natural way for someone with ADD to think of the time involved is by noticing what's being talked about, not how much time has passed. The content of the conversation is what counts. You might ask yourself, Did I finish what I had to say about that subject? Did I get the information I needed in order to understand the other person?

Though you may have thoroughly enjoyed your conversation, it probably wouldn't have occurred to you to ask yourself whether you wanted to pay the price of taking the time to have the conversation. Not thinking about time leaves you out of control, and that in turn causes stress.

Minutes and hours are artificial, arbitrary delineators of time. An ADD mind does not naturally think in these terms. Your difficulties with the way time is handled are natural for you, so don't kick yourself about it. There is nothing morally bad about not having a good sense of time. It's just different from people who do happen to be aware of the way time is measured.

The only aspect of time that many people with ADD are aware of is *now*, the moment in which we are living. Yesterday tends to be forgotten with its mistakes, and tomorrow never comes to mind. Is it any wonder, then, that you've been admonished, "Won't you ever learn from experience?" The continual innocence that many people with ADD have—ever hopeful that next time something will work out better—in part stems from their orientation to time.

Certainly, making plans for the future, even the immediate future, doesn't come to mind when you are absorbed in something that you want at the moment. You may be trying so hard to find something, that you fail to think of the long-term ramifications of what you're doing at the moment, so you're late again.

I'm not suggesting that you become obsessed with time to such an extent that you let your watch rule your life! But you need to have just enough awareness of time so that you can make a choice about whether to continue a conversation until you're naturally finished or to set an artificial time limit on it.

Time and Outwardly Expressive ADD

Hurrying from one thing to another, drawn to hundreds of distractions around you, you may appear to be a whirlwind to coworkers. Impulsively chasing whatever attracts you at the moment makes it very hard for you to get from point A to point B on time.

Are you cutting up, making jokes, and generally spending time getting people to like you, so much so that you forget about what time it is? Do your feelings of being blamed and criticized because you don't get to places in a timely manner make you want to give up even trying to be on time? If this sounds like you, you probably have a good deal of Outwardly Expressive ADD. As an "Active Entertainer," one of the last things that catches your attention is time passing. You're just not aware of it. Of course, if you're unaware of something, you can't do much about it. You need to become aware of the issue and develop a way of working on it that fits you comfortably.

When it comes to helping yourself feel better about things that seem to happen beyond your control, you could find yourself placing the blame on anyone or anything except yourself or using humor to diffuse your frustration. Your business lunch partner should have called you to confirm, for example for example, or the airlines have such stupid schedules! Anything to push the pain away from your inner feelings, which are masked behind a facade of blame or, sometimes, humor.

Time and Inwardly Directed ADD

Let's suppose you are more of an Inwardly Directed ADD. Appearing laid back, even easy going, you may find yourself daydreaming intensely, so much so that you lose track of time. Perhaps you started working on a project, and time slipped away. Creating, inventing, or talking with a friend or coworker grabs your attention a lot more readily than getting yourself prepared to attend a meeting, especially a meeting you think will be boring.

Though you never mean to put anyone else out, you could very well have forgotten a lunch date because you were so involved with that computer program that you forgot what day it was. Sure, this could happen to anyone once in a while, but the guilt you feel is all too familiar. So you blame yourself, wanting to disappear, hiding behind your computer screen all the more.

Others, though, are not likely to be aware of the guilt and blame you are already feeling. Their frequently heard statements, such as "Pay attention," "Quit goofing off," and "You're so irresponsible," only add to your unhappiness and frustration.

I recall a businessman who was responsible for making plane reservations to an out-of-town meeting. He also wanted to get some media coverage for his project. He was aware that he needed to make the reservations far enough in advance to get a good price, but he also knew that he was not likely to be able to set up the media interviews until closer to the time of his visit. With those two conflicting goals, his mind bounced back and forth, and he could not figure out when to make his reservation. Nor did it occur to him to ask for help, because he felt he *should* be able to solve the problem himself.

Unfortunately, he felt immobilized for so long that he failed to take advantage of good rates or call the radio and TV stations on time. Everyone on his work team ended up angry and disappointed in him. When asked why he hadn't made the reservations on time, he really couldn't remember. He knew he'd been thinking about it for a long time; he knew he wanted to do the right thing. But he couldn't recall that the reason for his nonaction was his immobilizing confusion.

Time and Highly Structured ADD

The "Conscientious Controller," the person with Highly Structured ADD, overcontrols situations. Had this person been faced with the plane reservation and media coverage dilemma, reservations would have been made three months in advance, and the media would have been contacted and pressed to fit his schedule. Accommodating the needs of the media would not be an issue for him. Rather, everyone else would be expected to accommodate him. He would phone his media contact almost daily to confirm the schedule and, before he ever arrived in town, be considered a pest and a nuisance.

Flexibility eludes people with Highly Structured ADD. If anything goes wrong—the schedule needs to be modified, for example— he is incapable of dealing calmly with the situation. If you have this form of ADD, you undoubtedly feel great anxiety, confusion, and frustration, though you may cover it with still more controlling and blaming exclamations.

"How could you do this to me?" you would ask. "You ought to have your organization under better control."

Scolding a lunch partner who had an urgent, last-minute change in plans, the Conscientious Controller might angrily say, "Well, this certainly cost me a day's work!" Compassion for the person needing to cancel usually is not a part of the picture. Is it any wonder people with Highly Structured ADD often create tension and stress in the workplace?

What the person with Highly Structured ADD is not saying is how anxious and out-of-control he is feeling inside. Those real feelings are masked by blaming, shaming behavior that puts others on the defensive. Often the person with this type of ADD has achieved a lot of power—he is good with details and quite precise—but he may use time as a weapon to control others, especially people who need something from him.

The person with Highly Structured ADD perceives time in such minute detail that every minute, even every second, may need to be accounted for. This person may not be easy to get along with in business, and relations with coworkers are often strained. If the Conscientious Controller has power or authority over others, time likely becomes a straitjacket to those around with everyone walking on eggshells for fear of misplacing a minute—much less an hour.

The Dreaded Deadline: April 15

Every job has its own deadlines and stresses, but there's one deadline we all have to face: April 15. As soon as we flip the calendar over to the new year, there it is, staring at us again. The ways we prepare for it—or don't prepare, as the case may be—vary from person to person. Here's how people with the different types of ADD and someone without ADD, all of whom want to make the deadline, would manage their time.

As January rolls around, Kevin, who has Outwardly Expressive ADD, is aware that it's time to start thinking about taxes, but he figures that April 15 is a long way off, and he has plenty of time.

"Honey, you take care of this stuff," he says to his wife. Not waiting for a response or even knowing whether she heard his request, he is on to more interesting things. As the W-2 and 1099 forms come in, Kevin tosses them in a pile on the desk. He never really thinks about preparing his taxes again until watching the late news on April 15, when he sees people lined up to mail their returns before midnight. Not only did neither his tax information get organized or a return get filed, but he didn't file an extension, either. Chagrined, not knowing how to solve the problem, and perhaps angry at the government, three years may pass without Kevin filing a return. If his wife asks him about it, he tells her not to worry. Kevin had every intention of filing his tax return; it just never happened.

Linda, who has Inwardly Directed ADD, also plans to file a return. On January 1 she also considers April 15 to be a long way off. If someone else in the family is available to do the job, she would be more than willing to turn the responsibility over to that person, but the issue of exactly who is taking that responsibility is never quite settled. As the forms come in, Linda says to herself, I should do something with this, but I don't know where to put it. I'll just leave it on my desk. And her desk is already piled high with various papers. Once during February and once in March, Linda thinks about her taxes, but she decides there's still plenty of time left before she needs to start preparing her return.

At the beginning of April, Linda sits down at her desk and thumbs through a few of the papers, deciding that it's time to get serious about her tax return. Just a few minutes after sitting down, she's interrupted by the phone ringing. A few minutes later, she feels sleepy. She thinks about her taxes again the next week and realizes she might need to file an extension. But she just doesn't know where to start. Feeling guilty and "stupid," Linda begins to feel overwhelmed, depressed, and hopeless about the whole business. She keeps meaning to file a return, but instead she turns on the TV. When April 15 comes around, Linda, like Kevin, hasn't prepared a return or an extension.

In contrast to these two, Angie, who is Highly Structured ADD, takes immediate and total control of her tax situation—beginning January 1. She knows she can do a better job of preparing a tax return than anyone else. She sets up an organizer labeled with slots for each type of form she expects to receive. She marks dates on her calendar to remind her to collect her data and turn it over to her accountant. As each form and slip of paper arrives, she labels and sorts it. She reads and labels all receipts.

Problems come for Angie, however, when one of her employers types her social security number incorrectly on a W-2 form. This throws her whole plan and entire schedule off course. She calls the woman responsible and screams at her over the phone. After all, this terrible mistake and the need to have this form retyped has upset Angie's whole plan. She calls the woman twice a day to ask about the form until the corrected copy arrives in the mail. Then Angie's printer runs out of ink. She becomes obsessed with getting to the store to buy a new cartridge. When she replaces the cartridge and begins working on her return, no one in the house is allowed to do anything that might interrupt her.

Angie just might get her tax return finished or an extension filed on time. Chances are, though, she alienated quite a few people in the process, everyone from her children, to the personnel officer at her work-place, to the cashier at the office supply store. Just being around Angie has been stressful for her family and coworkers. They are all glad that April 15 has passed. They dread its next arrival.

Rodney, who does not have ADD, checks his calendar in January and is aware that April 15 isn't too far away. He realizes that tax forms will be arriving soon in the mail and decides to keep them in his lower desk drawer. He thinks about a preliminary timetable for completing his tax return, and he and his wife discuss who is going to do which part of the tax preparation work.

In mid-February, Rodney makes sure that all the required forms have been received. He decides to sacrifice one weekend to work on his tax return in March. If a delay occurs, or a W-2 has been printed incorrectly, Rodney makes sure to fix the problem and makes a readjustment to his fairly loose schedule. If he sees that the return cannot be prepared on time, he files an extension by the appropriate deadline. No one really enjoys preparing their taxes, but for Rodney, major stress and failure are not a part of this picture.

Time-Related Conflicts between People with Different Types of ADD

Since people with different types of ADD perceive and work with time issues differently, it's predictable that there will be some conflicts when they find themselves together in the workplace.

For example, one of the ways people with Outwardly Expressive ADD learn to manage time and make use of their ADD is by waiting until the last minute to prepare for whatever they are doing. When a speaker with this type of ADD begins to study information for her speech topic the day before leaving for a presentation, the uninformed person could wonder how such an irresponsible speaker could possibly have been chosen to give the keynote address. What isn't apparent is the added drive and high level of focus this last-minute pressure provides for the speaker.

Imagine a person with Outwardly Expressive ADD sharing responsibility for a workshop presentation with someone who has Highly Structured ADD. The person with Highly Structured ADD would begin preparations months ahead, researching and writing his presentation, reading it aloud, rewriting, practicing his delivery, and taking note cards to the opening session with everything he ever learned written down. He would expect his partner to do the same, but the person with Outwardly Expressive ADD might have already begun to feel burned out by his coworker's obsession with preparation. Exasperated when asked to make an outline and turn it in weeks ahead of time, the person with Outwardly Expressive ADD would probably either refuse to do the outline or, feeling a lot of resentment, do a sloppy job. Although he would most likely arrive at the workshop without any written notes, he would probably be able to talk spontaneously on any subject in his field. Imagine the consternation of the person with Highly Structured ADD when he enters the conference room and his coworker asks, "What are we presenting on today?"

For many people with Outwardly Expressive ADD, a long period of detailed preparation can take the edge off their creativity, and they can end up making poorer presentations than they would have made without extensive preparation. The sharpness associated with a spontaneous performance by a talented stand-up comic, entertainer, or extemporaneous speaker is usually dulled with practice.

Although it is difficult for a person with Outwardly Expressive ADD and one with Highly Structured ADD to understand one another, they each must respect the other's style and methods for preparing a successful professional presentation. This kind of trust comes only with experience and their eventual understanding that they are simply wired differently from each other.

This same type of conflict occurs when coaches do not understand that different athletes, some of whom have ADD, prepare differently for performance on the field. One athlete may be praised because she gives 110 percent all the time, practicing hard and playing hard. By contrast, the athlete who doesn't "get up" for practice but performs spectacularly on the playing field during the contest, may be seen as lazy, irresponsible, and a poor example for other players.

In reality, each athlete may be preparing in exactly the right way, according to his or her own internal wiring. But many a player has been cut or chastised for not pushing himself or herself to the limit during practice. Some very talented, skillful teams may be shortchanging themselves because of a lack of understanding of the variety of ways in which people learn.

This is true of any job or profession. The trick is to honestly assess yourself and proceed in the manner that fits best. Each of us needs to honor our coworkers' styles of preparation—especially when the coworkers' performances are successful—asking questions when we don't understand but never automatically criticizing because the others' ways are different.

Time-Related Conflicts between ADD and Non-ADD Coworkers

When ADD and non-ADD coworkers share an assignment or project, there is bound to be conflict in time management unless the coworkers have discussed the issues and made an effort to understand each other's style of planning and working.

For example, consider coworkers who need to attend an out-of-town meeting and decide to travel together. Joe, who has ADD, volunteers to pick up Caroline, who does not have ADD, to drive to the airport together. Joe suggests a pickup time that will keep waiting time at the airport to a minimum, because he hates the idea of having to just sit and wait for the plane for any extended period of time. That makes Caroline nervous; she's concerned they won't be arriving at the airport early enough. But Joe assures her, "All will be well. I do it all the time." Caroline agrees to Joe's suggestion.

Unfortunately, Joe arrives at Caroline's house later than he had planned, so he speeds down the road trying to make up the lost time. During the drive Caroline is trying to figure out the best way to manage the bags at the airport to save time, and she becomes increasingly apprehensive about missing the flight.

If the close-in parking lot is full, or anything else happens to further delay the pair, there's a good chance they'll miss the plane. Because of this incident, angry words or bottled-up resentment could affect their working relationship throughout the trip and could even potentially cost them the client they were traveling to meet. If they miss the plane, the client might question the judgment of the firm employing the person with ADD.

Joe never meant for any of this to happen. He was just trying to schedule the drive to the airport so that he could avoid a long wait for the plane. However, he may have endangered an important working relationship because of his inability to properly organize his time.

What Can You Do to Help Yourself Manage Time?

Setting clocks ahead, a favorite suggestion of people who do not have ADD, does not work for those with ADD. As one woman so succinctly put it, "I know I set them ahead so my mind adjusts for the difference. I know it's a game."

Getting ready earlier than normal doesn't work either. "That simply gives me more time to get distracted before it's time to leave," says another person with ADD.

So, what does work? If you have trouble keeping track of time, the first thing you have to do is make a commitment to work on remedying a problem that seems hopeless to you. If you're willing to make that commitment, give yourself permission to use whatever you need to help yourself.

If you like gadgets, mechanical aids may serve you well. Consider three forms:

- **Auditory aids** such as buzzers or alarms that can be found on watches, clocks, and timers. These are good if you are sensitive and responsive to sound. When you hear the buzzer, you must be willing to act immediately, or you will become distracted by other sounds and forget that your alarm went off.

- **Visual aids** include digital timers that you can set for however much time you have left to complete a specific activity. Again, you must be willing to immediately stop, change, or move when the timer hits zero. Place it right in front of you. Even the old-fashioned three-minute egg timer works if you have a visual orientation to the world. Also, you could post notes in obvious places to remind yourself of when you've decided to start or stop a certain task.

- **Kinesthetic aids** set up a vibration that cues you at the set time, or you may set one to vibrate periodically to nudge you to pay attention. This is good for people whose strongest sense is touch.

Don't hesitate to ask people to help you stay on task or give you a reminder to get going. If you do form this type of partnership with a coworker, friend, or family member, be sure you respond to the reminder and thank the person. This is very different from the feelings you have when anyone else constantly reminds you to stay busy someone you haven't asked for help. That usually feels like nagging.

You might consider making a trade-off with your boss. If you need support from other staff in order to accomplish your work on time, but having that support is not officially in your job description, you might ask your boss to provide you with support staff in exchange for increased productivity. For example, maybe management would provide one hour of an administrative assistant's time to help you with your paperwork per an agreed-upon dollar volume of business that you bring to the company. If that sounds like a solution that might work for you, don't worry about suggesting it to your boss. After all, the company and you will both benefit from your increased productivity.

I've found that giving rewards for improved time management is important. When a task is hard—and for people with ADD, learning to manage time in the workplace is hard—we need all the help we can get. So, each time you meet a time commitment or improve your timing, reward yourself with a mental or physical treat. Your treat can be as simple as a voice in your head that says, Good job. I'm proud of you. It can be a compliment from a partner, a walk in the sunshine, or even a favorite piece of chocolate.

Until you have fairly good control over your time, you may want to spare yourself and others from your time-management difficulties by not going places with them. Take two cars and say, "Go on ahead and start if I'm not there." You need to pay the consequences yourself as much as possible for being late, rather than making your coworkers pay them. The idea here is to stop fooling yourself, or someone else, that you can accomplish something you haven't yet mastered.

Though, like Joe in the airport drive example, your intentions are good, you need to take time to build the skills that don't come naturally to you. I find that I have to periodically remind myself to stay on schedule. If I don't, or if I'm tired, my timing gets sloppy, and I revert back to not getting places on time, misjudging how long it will take me to do a particular task, or becoming oblivious to time altogether. The whole trick is to raise your level of consciousness about time so you pay attention to it. But be sure it's you who is motivating you—not someone else nagging you.

The Physical Organization of Your Workspace

When you decided to sit down and read just now, did you have trouble finding this book? How much time did you spend looking for it? When you stop reading and have to move on to another activity, where will you put the book?

Do you usually spend quite a bit of time looking for the tools and materials you need to begin an activity, whether they're your socks and shoes in the morning or a specific drafting pencil? At work do your tools and materials get lost because there's not a specific place for them? If so, you probably already know that's bad for your job and bad for business—and it's an issue that many people with ADD face. Can you do anything about it? Yes. Even though keeping track of the many pieces of paper, tools, and details of work may not be natural for you, you can learn to become more organized yourself, or you can get help.

You are not a bad person because you misplace or lose things. Even people who do not have ADD spend some time looking for things that aren't where they thought they would be. For someone with ADD, though, the frequency and magnitude of lack of organization is greater.

One woman said to me, "Everyone has some room or drawer in

their house that they've needed to get to for years and years, but they don't because it is just too overwhelming. My whole life is that way."

For many people with ADD, there are so many things to keep track of that it is overwhelming to consider *getting* organized, much less *staying* organized. The exceptions are people who have Highly Structured ADD, who are usually very organized. In fact, they are usually overorganized and find it difficult to cope if anything comes along that doesn't fit precisely into their organizational schemes.

The Consequences of Being Disorganized

It is important to understand that neatness is often considered a moral issue in our culture, but there is no instrinsic reason for it to be that way. Nevertheless, the fact that it is a moral issue only compounds the sense of failure that many people with ADD feel. When you try again and again to organize your desk, your office, or your workroom, and again and again you can't seem to find what you need, the feeling you have is one of intense personal failure, as if your behavior were somehow going against the moral structure of society.

It's not that you weren't taught to be neat or that you don't want to be neat. It's just that your brain is wired differently from someone who does not have ADD. Your brain doesn't allow you to look at pieces of paper, tools, and other things in an orderly manner. For you, the world is just not made up of slots, folders, or straight lines.

As someone with ADD, what you pay attention to is different from what those who are orderly do. You may find that you are paying more attention to the function of a tool than where to keep it. You may respond to what's written on the page in your hand more than where you should file that page. You could be distracted as you're on your way to putting something away, and it just gets left, probably in the place nearest to where you were standing when you needed to use that hand for something else.

Because placing things in prearranged places is not natural for you, trying to figure out what to do with a particular paper or tool may take a lot of time—so much time that you forget what you're doing, quit looking for a place to put the item because you feel confused, or throw it down on a pile out of frustration.

As you already know, the implications of this lack of organization for business are very serious. You spend too much of your valuable time just trying to find things. As a result, you can miss business opportunities and leads. You delay other work that needs to be accomplished while you're looking for the tools you need. Even money, or records of money, can be lost, and you may never find them. In addition, your slovenly desk may make people think you can't be trusted to do a good job. That analysis might be completely untrue, but first impressions often do win or lose deals.

Overwhelmed by Business Cards?

Let's start formulating some ideas for getting organized by looking at the piece of paper that often accompanies your meeting a new business person: the business card. These little bitty pieces of paper are really difficult to keep track of, even for someone who doesn't have ADD. But for someone with ADD, the tens or hundreds of them you might acquire in a year can add up to a nightmare.

Joanna, a charismatic, successful professional who has ADD, once told me how frustrated she becomes when she makes business contacts. She exchanges business cards with people and has every intention of following up on the contact, but then has no idea how to keep track of the cards. Days or months later, if Joanna finds a business card in her pocket, she remembers there was some reason she took the card, but that reason is long gone. Because she is better with the social aspects of meeting people than with the business angle of keeping track of her contacts—which she finds very boring—she forgets the networking ideas that were triggered when she was in the middle of the conversation, even though she found those ideas exciting at the time. So, instead of being able to use the business leads, she often loses them.

Even if Joanna does get the business cards out of her jacket pocket or purse and into the office, she can't figure out how to organize them. Knowing that she won't remember the stranger's name, she tries to organize the cards by category. But she becomes frustrated and gives up when she can't decide which category to put a particular card in. She has tried having one file specifically for business cards, but the file became just a large heap of cards, and she wasn't able to find anything in it. Overwhelmed, Joanna doesn't do anything at all with her business cards—losing them and the contacts.

Though Messy, Do You Really Know Where Things Are?

Some people with ADD may be able to look at a pile of paper on their desks and go right to the piece of paper they need. Ever known a mechanic whose tool box looked worse that a three-year-old's toy box, but the fellow could dig his hand down in the heap, pulling out the exact tool he was looking for? Was that accidental or just plain luck? No! It's just that the filing system these people use is different from the regularly recognized, generally accepted, clean-cut style. Most people with ADD have an inner sense of knowing what works well for them; sometimes it's called intuition. And it works!

It may be that the mechanic knew he put his tool down on the left side of his box when he was working earlier. He remembers also putting several other tools in his box on that side and figures that the first tool is buried about three tools deep. He goes unerringly to the tool because he measures things by a sense of depth and direction. Maybe the salesman, whose desk is heaped high with orders and invoices, knows that unfinished business is placed in a certain area on the desk, whereas completed sales paperwork, to be filed, is somewhere else. So the problem may not be that the item can't be found; the problem is that other people—and, by now, the person with ADD, too—have come to believe that there is something wrong with having a messy workspace. Even if the messy workspace is functioning just fine for its owner, they still believe messy is "bad." From that attitude, people with ADD take on a tremendous amount of guilt, guilt that is learned when you think you're doing something wrong.

You need to determine whether to feel guilty or not. First check to see whether you actually have a problem in this area or only think you do. Ask yourself, Can I still function well with my messiness, or not?

You may be surprised to find out that many people with ADD share this problem. People who don't have ADD are often shocked at how frequently those of us with ADD can find things regardless of the state of the mess. Conversely, having things in a neat order does not guarantee that people with ADD will find what they are looking for. In fact, I have probably lost more things that were filed in some logical category than I've lost by having them in an unnamed or unmarked stack near my workplace.

Keeping Track of Things

All the wonderful filing systems in the world will not help you stay organized if you don't think the same way as the system is set up. To keep track of papers, I'd suggest coming up with the categories yourself, even if someone else helps you put the things in order. I strongly suggest that you hire someone to help you set the organization up initially, even if your "hiring" involves cutting a deal with your spouse to trade filing for yard work. It takes some of the pressure off if all you have to do is think up categories. It also helps if the person assisting you stays around because, if you forget the category, perhaps that person will recall it.

Before investing in expensive filing systems for your shop or office, try a small sample and see if you would actually use it. You would be a lot better off with cardboard boxes lined up on the floor against the wall—labeled "future work," "work in progress," "completed work," and "I don't know what to do with this stuff"—than with a sophisticated filing system that just doesn't work for you.

One example of sorting that works well for many people came from a hardware store owner, Sam, whose desk in the back room of the store had not been touched for twenty years. He had no idea where to start. In a training group to help him deal with organization, he was assigned a partner, T.J., whose job it was to pick the pieces of paper off the desk one at a time, then ask him which of three piles to put them in. They agreed in advance to do only one fourth of the desk at their first meeting, so that the task wouldn't seem quite as overwhelming.

Sam and T.J. met at the appointed time. T.J. divided the desk into quarters using masking tape, and Sam decided which quarter to start with. Three trash bags were laid out on the floor. One was marked, "I can't live without this." The second read, "Throw it away." And the third, "I don't know what to do with this stuff but might need to keep it."

The first quarter of Sam's desk was cleared in less than an hour. He felt so good that the next morning he finished the whole desk. Then he asked T.J. to help him with the "I don't know" stack. It was just a matter of someone asking him questions about the individual pieces.

Sam enjoyed the social aspect of the project, too. That helped him focus his attention and even enjoy a situation that otherwise would have been very uncomfortable for him.

One of the difficulties that overwhelm people with ADD is that they try to do too much at one time, lumping together several steps of a project that should really be done separately. For example, you might need to keep financial records but might avoid the task because you don't know where to file the information after it's collected. Instead of considering the entire project, start by just making a pile of financial records. It's another job entirely to actually divide them by year or put them into categories, such as "personal" and "business." To keep everything in order, you might need to have someone help you out on a regular basis either monthly or, for example, when the stack gets two inches high. Choose what feels best to you.

Many of us keep baskets and boxes to hold things like bills and receipts until it's time to work on them. Sometimes that's just a way to avoid getting organized, which you have to do eventually. So go ahead and face it, but do it with help and rewards afterwards. Don't bury your head in the sand!

"Sticky notes" and other reminders of all kinds are helpful. Post them on the bathroom mirrors, across doorjambs and on the steering wheel of your car. If you like color, use it: as dividers, to catch your attention, and to associate with certain categories.

I know one college student who is ADD who made a daily reminder chart, marking time periods with colors for each type of activity he had to do. For example, the times when he was to go to class were marked with blue. Study time was marked with yellow. Times marked in red reminded him that it was time to go to his job. Meal times were marked in white. And TV-watching time was colored green.

All he had to do was glance at his daily chart, posted on his notebook, and he instantly knew what he needed to do next. This helped him get where he needed to go on time until he became habituated to his schedule for the semester. At the beginning of each new semester, this type of chart was a necessity for him—and he knew it.

If you can learn to use a date book, do so, but be sure to be patient with yourself. Don't expect to get it right immediately. It may take a young adult a year to get in the habit of consulting his date book regularly. If the idea of using one is appealing to you, though, begin using it. You might find that a partner reminding you to check it helps turn its use into a habit. When you fall off the track, just pick yourself up and start over.

Some people with ADD prefer to use blank sheets of paper every day, making notes of what needs to be done and crossing those items off the list as the tasks are completed.

What is important is to know that there is not *one* right way to do things, but that you need to find *your* way. Above all, give yourself permission to turn a lot of your organizational tasks over to others, with their permission, of course. Your talents can be better used in other ways than struggling to do something that is not natural or is exceedingly hard for you.

You're a good person whether you can keep track of your own things or not. What is important is that what needs to be organized is organized, not who does the job.

Project Management

Almost everything we do takes some long-term planning and management strategies. The need for project management skills is just a fact of life if projects are to be done efficiently or even completed at all. In the workplace, projects range from moving an office or a shop to preparing an annual report. No matter what kind of work you do, you have to deal with the planning of long-term projects at some time. Whether it's writing a book, designing a fashion show, changing out the engine in a car, or hosting a convention for your profession, they all require project management skills.

Many people with ADD do not realize the amount of time and effort that non-ADD people put into long-term planning. By nature, people with ADD tend to approach all situations spontaneously. The thought of breaking a project down into manageable bits just doesn't readily occur to us.

The truth is, to manage any project, there is a set of skills that is required: working with deadlines, keeping track of what's being done, organizing tools and materials, and communicating what's needed and what's being accomplished. That's a lot of organization! It's probably the ultimate organizational challenge for people with ADD.

To see how important project management skills are at work, and how people with differing types of ADD might deal with these issues, let's look at the following four examples. Let's assume that each of the four persons we're focusing on owns part of a small company that manufactures picture frames. A local decorator has just placed the largest order the company has ever had. She needs fifty frames of specific shapes and colors within four weeks.

Adam, a Business Owner with Outwardly Expressive ADD

Adam shouts enthusiastically and jumps around with joy when the order comes in from the decorator. He tells everyone he comes in contact with about his great luck in landing this job. He tells people that he's going to use the money he makes on this job to upgrade his business. In his mind he has already completed the job, and he sees himself and the business as highly successful. This is the break he's been waiting for.

As Adam talks with people, he continues to find new ways to utilize his projected profits. He's very enthusiastic about all the ways he can parlay the money he earns into an ever more successful business for him and his partner. It makes him feel good to share such profits.

The day after receiving the job, Adam thinks about the fact that he is going to have to order some supplies, but he continues to spend his time considering his business expansion plans—plans that are built on the other jobs he is now sure will come his way. He's not worried about getting the supply order turned in; after all, he has four weeks.

Late on Friday of the first week, Adam realizes he still hasn't ordered the mat board he needs, but he realizes it will have to wait until Monday. On Monday morning he picks up the phone to order the supplies. Then he realizes he hasn't calculated the exact amount of board he'll need of each color, so he estimates the amounts he'll need as he places the order. In the past he's been pretty good at estimating the supplies he'll need, but he doesn't consider that he's never had an order this large before.

At the end of the second week, the decorator calls to see how the project is going. Adam tells her everything is fine and thanks her again for her order. He hasn't heard back from the company he ordered the supplies from, but he assumes everything is coming along fine. For a moment, he gets a queasy feeling in his stomach but immediately tells himself everything is okay.

Later that day Adam calls the company to check on the mat board. The mats are not ready, and there's a problem with the order. He hadn't mentioned any deadline to the supplier, so they hadn't called to tell him of the problem. Adam yells at the clerk, then apologizes, realizing that he'll have to do business with this company again in the future.

Within a few days Adam's happiness turns to anxiety. He begins to have trouble sleeping at night, worrying that the job won't be completed in time. He is irritable in the shop and talks angrily about the inadequacies of the companies he's dealing with.

Finally, with less than a week left, his materials have arrived, and he's ready to begin work. Immediately he begins yelling at the employees, "Where are my tools? Who's been using my tools? My knives are dull!" It had never occurred to Adam to check his tools ahead of time.

For the last few days before his deadline, Adam works nonstop day and night. In the frenzy to finish the job on time, he forgets his wife's birthday and his daughter's dance recital. His family is mad at him, his coworkers are disgusted with him, and he doesn't understand why everyone is being so mean just when he has so much work to do. After all, he's doing the best he can under adverse circumstances!

Even if Adam completes the order on time, the frames are likely to be inferior to the ones he builds one at a time because he is rushed. The decorator might like his creativity and work on an individual frame, but she will probably not be happy with his efforts at mass production. She probably won't give him any more large orders. Dejected, Adam reacts by saying that he never needed her business, anyway.

Adam never did have a strategic, long-term plan for producing those frames. He did try the best he could, but he didn't realize that manufacturing fifty frames is a completely different process from manufacturing one frame. He had no concept of how to break up the four weeks' time—and the project—into manageable bits.

Sasha, a Business Owner with Inwardly Directed ADD

The creative opportunity Sasha has been looking for arrives when she receives an order for fifty picture frames. She is thrilled. Sasha loves to design frames; since becoming a partner in this framing business, she has never been happier.

The day she receives the order, hundreds of ideas play through her mind: materials, colors, mat board styles, and the little extras she knows will make her frames stand out. Consumed in a wonderland of delight, several days go by before Sasha realizes she'd better narrow her options and order some materials. Sasha tries to figure out how much material she'll need, but she soon realizes that ordering for fifty frames is much more complicated than ordering materials for just a few. The more she tries to figure out what she needs, the more confused she becomes. Eventually, she takes the step and places her order for materials.

Sasha wants to begin work when the materials arrive, but she can't seem to keep track of her tools. When she does find the right tool, she is indecisive about the design of the frames. Should she make this change? Should she make that change? More time goes by, and she experiments with the frames and daydreams about artistic possibilities of so many frames.

As her deadline approaches, Sasha begins to get depressed, fearing she might not be able to finish the project on time. Her depression causes her to work even slower. She spends a lot of time feeling guilty and blaming herself for her inability to complete the project. She doesn't sleep well, and the circles under her eyes deepen. She's already decided that she's failed—and that slows her down even more. Feeling helpless and sure she can't do anything right, Sasha sits and stares out the window. The only thing she can think about is quitting the business.

Sasha didn't think about making a project plan initially, nor did she have any way to monitor her progress. And she didn't think to ask for help along the way. Her coworkers, in the meantime, were wondering why Sasha, such a talented artist, wouldn't talk to them. From their perspective, she was doing a beautiful job. True, she was slow, but what she did looked great and was extremely creative. They couldn't figure out why she quit.

Celia, a Business Owner with Highly Structured ADD

Celia began making her plans the minute she hung up the phone from the decorator. That same day, she counted her inventory of mat boards, figured out what colors and textures to use, and made notes to check on some new materials she had heard about.

By the second day, Celia had her schedule planned out for each day for the coming month, and she had written down every detail in her calendar. She also placed her mat board order and checked with the company about deadlines. By the end of the day, she had mailed letters to the decorator, her partner, and the mat board company summarizing their phone conversations. She placed a copy of each letter in her new file, which was marked with the project deadline.

Each day, Celia checks her calendar, asks her employees about their progress, counts her tools, chastises anyone who has used one of her tools, and generally watches every move her employees make. She is demanding, possessive, and very controlling in her management of the project.

Though Celia is dedicated to getting the job done, she creates a lot of bad feelings among her employees and coworkers. She hounds the mat board company, talking incessantly about her order. And she calls the decorator almost daily, updating her on the order's progress.

As the deadline nears, Celia becomes more and more irritable and controlling. If someone interrupts her or moves a tool, she screams at him. If someone uses a tool for the wrong material, she falls apart.

A perfectionist, Celia has little ability to be flexible or accommodate any change in plans. When the mat board company can't get one brand but finds a substitute that is comparable, she yells at them, too. Celia is fixated on the plans she has made and has a hard time moving on to continue her work in a new direction.

Celia thinks she is the only one contributing to the job; no one else's role in valued. Though she will probably get the job done correctly and on time, she leaves a lot of bad feelings and hurt in her wake. Chances are that the decorator will like the picture frames but wouldn't choose to work with Celia again because of her personality.

Juan, a Non-ADD Business Owner

Juan is overjoyed at receiving the order for fifty frames. It's the largest order his company has ever received. He calls his partner and suggests they go out to dinner to celebrate and make some preliminary plans for handling personnel, ordering, and supervision. At dinner they discuss each of the business issues briefly and agree to complete the planning the next day. Then they enjoy the rest of the evening free of shoptalk.

The next day Juan spends some time visualizing the creative aspects of the project: how he'd like the frames to look and how he could make them uniquely fit the decorator's needs. Then Juan asks himself some questions and jots down the answers in a small notebook:

- How long will it take me to make one frame?
- Will it take me the same amount of time per frame to make fifty?
- Can I accomplish the work by the deadline by myself, or do I need help?
- If I need help, what kind of help do I need? How much help? And where can I find it?
- What materials and tools will I need?
- Do I have them on hand, or do I need to order them?
- How long will it take to get the supplies?
- What companies should I order supplies from?
- How often do I need to check back with them?

Then Juan takes out his calendar and marks the dates by which materials need to be ordered and construction begun. He also jots himself a note to call the decorator once or twice during the month to let her know how things are progressing. If he's having any problems with production, he can let her know what's going on and make any necessary and appropriate changes in deadlines or products.

He completely clears his calendar during the last week of production to make sure he will be available to handle any last-minute problems that might come up. Even non-ADD people who are mostly organized have "crunch" times; the difference may be that accommodation is made ahead of time to allow for them. People who do not have ADD usually don't come unglued during crunches or ignore them, either. Rather, such periods are part of the organizational plan.

The decorator probably finds working with Juan satisfying. He doesn't take a lot of her time, and her doesn't let her down; he just gets the job done. His artistry is not lost because of organizational problems. This decorator is likely to consider working with Juan again.

Tips for Project Management

If it doesn't come naturally for you to break a large project into doable parts, don't panic. It doesn't have to be a nightmare. Practice does help a person learn what steps to take and how to accomplish tasks one at a time.

If you need help learning how to break the project down into manageable parts, do not hesitate to ask for it. But be careful: if the suggestions you're getting still don't seem to make the project manageable, say so. The person helping you must search, with your input, to find alternative ways to do the job.

If you are working with a helper and feel that familiar sick feeling in your stomach that comes from being overwhelmed, keep working to find an alternative plan so you can be comfortable. Don't just turn your mind off, although that may seem an attractive escape from the confusion and discomfort.

Try not to put your energy into crying, flying into a rage, or running away. Try to keep focusing your energy on developing an alternate plan that will work for you. Take it slowly, check each step to make sure that you and your helper are still thinking along the same lines, and pay close attention to understanding what is being said. Tell your helper to stop as soon as you begin to feel a sense of information overload. Back up and take it piece by piece again, or continue the discussions at a later date.

You can also participate in ADD training workshops that address issues of project management. Sometimes these groups, with the help of a leader, simulate breaking projects down into manageable chunks. That would give you a chance to practice project management without the consequences of actually having to do the work. The people with ADD who participate in these workshops usually find out that they have some very valid ideas about managing projects. Each person, however, must learn what works best for him or her and still gets the job done.

If you don't participate in a local group, you can do an exercise by yourself that would simulate the experience of the group. Make up a project and a deadline. Keep it fairly simple, but make sure it has several steps. Then write down these questions, and the answers to them:

- What do I need to accomplish?
- How much time do I have to complete the job?
- Do I need help?

Next ask yourself what steps are involved in the project. If you can't figure out which one needs to come first, jot down all the steps, then read them through carefully a few times. You will be able to see which step is the one that really needs to be done first.

Be sure to divide the project into *many* small steps, so that each step can be completed in a reasonable amount of time, and you can check it off your list. That will help you from feeling overwhelmed. Then apply a preliminary timetable to your project. It can be loose, but pin it down as much as possible. Always mark your schedule on your calendar in pencil so you can easily modify it as the project moves forward.

Be sure to weave some extra time into your schedule for unexpected events. If you are prepared in advance for the fact that something unexpected *will* come up—even though you can't imagine what that could be right now—your schedule will be able to accommodate it.

Then go back over your whole plan again and see whether any of the steps you've created can be broken down further or be made more manageable. Know yourself and be honest when deciding how much you can tackle at once. Be sure to plan in breaks and rewards.

You may find that talking about your project with someone helps you. Do it. Teamwork on the job, fortunately, is getting much more popular. It's a smart way to utilize diverse talents. Your best bet is to talk about your project only with people who are positive, draw you out, or have suggestions that make your work better. Avoid critics and devil's advocates.

Let your coworkers know about the plan you've developed for managing your project. Let them know when you will be working on the project and at what times you can and cannot be interrupted. Don't be afraid to ask for help at any time along the way, especially with the structuring of the project. You can go back and do the work once it's structured.

Be nice to yourself. Don't expect perfection the first time you try this. It may take many projects until you become really expert at breaking them down into manageable pieces, but you will find that you've improved even from the first to the second project you tackle. You will succeed either alone or with an organizational partner.

If you have Outwardly Expressive or Inwardly Directed ADD, you probably won't make your living by organizing projects, but you *can* lose your fear of tackling any organizational task. You can become responsible for seeing that organization happens, and you can contribute to its accomplishment.

If you have Highly Structured ADD, you might well make your living organizing projects or working within a highly organized structure. Just don't judge others who do not share your interests or abilities. Appreciate your opposites for what they have to offer. Then join forces.

It's teamwork that gets the job done.

4

Communication Skills in the Workplace

Jeffrey bounded into his boss's office one day, enthusiastic but with a deadly serious expression on his face. Not taking the time to ask whether or not he was interrupting, he launched into a monologue about the merits of a particular computer software package he had just purchased that "would help *anyone* get organized." His boss was taken aback by Jeffrey's interruption, but he listened politely for a few minutes.

"You need to get this," Jeffrey said. "Everyone in the office needs to have this program on their computer."

Though it was difficult to get a word in edgewise, his boss finally interrupted in the middle of a sentence and said, "Jeffrey, I'm glad you've found something that helps *you*."

Jeffrey, who is ADD, never missed a beat. "You've got to get it. It will help you," he counseled his boss.

At that point his boss began to feel pressed, but he stayed composed and said, "Jeffrey, I'm glad you like it, but it's not something I'm interested in using personally."

"It only takes fifteen minutes at the beginning and end of each day, and it will get your life totally under control," Jeffrey continued. "I mean it. This is great. You've got to see it."

By failing to acknowledge the boss's comment and by continuing to press his point, Jeffrey was well on his way to alienating his boss.

"I'm not interested in a program like that, Jeffrey," his boss said. "It's just not for me, but I'm sure it has value for many people."

Jeffrey made another comment about the value of the program, then told his boss where he could purchase it and how much it cost.

By then, his boss was irritated and just wanted Jeffrey out of his office. Firmly, even a little harshly, his boss said, "Thank you, Jeffrey. I have to go on to other things now. Good-bye." He picked up his phone to make a call.

His boss felt irritated and discounted. Jeffrey hadn't heard a word he'd said. Jeffrey was so self-absorbed that there didn't even seem to be any interest on Jeffrey's part to hear what his boss was saying. His boss, on the other hand, was expecting a two-way conversation in which Jeffrey would respond to his input, but that certainly didn't happen. From this conversation, his boss began to have great doubts about Jeffrey's competency.

In his hyperfocused, compulsive sales pitch, Jeffrey failed the first rule of communication: to watch the other person and listen to his response to what is being said. His boss learned something too: just because you are talking to someone doesn't mean he is listening.

In a real dialogue, which is what Jeffrey's boss would have preferred, the participants attempt to check out whether or not "true" communication has occurred: whether the receiver has heard the message that the sender planned to communicate. Dialogue takes time. It involves each person contributing equal parts of listening and speaking, including nonverbal gestures and behaviors that support what is being said. It takes a number of interchanges to check and clarify the intent of each person.

It takes a lot of sustained attention to engage in quality dialogue. That's one of the reasons people with ADD often have difficulty with communication. People with ADD may talk a lot, but talking rapidly or constantly does not guarantee good communication. Verbal hyperactivity is a symptom of all three types of ADD, and it does not lead to good communication in the workplace or anywhere else. Instead of good communication, this chattering is really an expenditure of words that is used to drain off the extra energy the person has inside.

People with Highly Structured ADD are often compulsive talkers, not hearing, or even really looking for, a response. Rather, that type of person talks as if a phonograph needle had become stuck, frequently making the same point over and over and over in a serious and intense manner.

Many of the hidden difficulties that come from having ADD show up in the workplace as problems with communication. People with ADD frequently have problems with speaking impulsively, interrupting, not telling the truth, communicating poorly in writing, and not listening effectively, especially if the persons they are listening to speak slowly.

On the other hand, ADD can provide a positive edge for people who have learned to use language effectively. Many times, the ability to "b.s." one's way through school translates into good work skills. The verbal comedic performances of someone with Outwardly Expressive ADD can be entertaining. Also, charismatic speaking energized by ADD can capture the listener's attention and be effective in educating audiences.

ADD can also be an advantage when it comes to nonverbal communication; many people with ADD can read others' nonverbal communication like a book. The up side of this ability is that people with ADD are well suited to careers that benefit from a strong sense of intuition, such as a teacher or family therapist. The down side is that the person may jump to the wrong conclusions because of their beliefs or counter what they don't like with their own nonverbal gestures and grimaces. Nonverbal communication is powerful. Entire business deals have been made or broken without a word being spoken.

"But I Assumed . . ."

All communication is based on certain assumptions made by the speaker and the listener. The difficulty for people with ADD is this: people who are not ADD often make one set of assumptions about communication, and people who are ADD often make a completely different set. That disparity creates the basis of a great deal of misunderstanding in the workplace.

The most basic assumption people make is that the person with whom you are speaking is in fact listening to you. As we saw Jeffrey's boss learn, though, that might not always be the case, especially if the person you're speaking with has ADD. It takes a lot of energy to really focus on, concentrate on, and listen to what's being said. And that is very difficult if you are ADD.

For example, Marian, who is ADD, found her mind drifting constantly as her coworker was explaining a new public relations pitch she'd devised. Marian wanted to listen. She even wanted to take part in the campaign. But after a few minutes, she realized she had missed some vital points of information. What could she do? She continued to listen, as intently as she could, hoping that the information would be repeated. Her coworker, however, assumed Marian had heard her the first time and that she would ask a question if something came up she didn't understand. The coworker didn't understand the fundamental problem: it wasn't that Marian was confused about a particular issue—it was that Marian had never received the information in the first place, because she had tuned out.

Of course, it would have been best if Marian could have acknowledged the communication lapses and simply said, "I'm sorry. My mind drifted off. Would you repeat what you said?"

If your coworkers know you have ADD and understand what that means, they might realize how much difficulty you have with sustained listening. Once they are aware of that, they will know they cannot automatically assume you have heard *and* processed what was said. It would be in their best interests to check with you and ask directly whether or not you heard their comments or directions. Then you must answer honestly.

People who do not have ADD often assume that their way of doing things is right and everyone else's—particularly the way of those with ADD—is wrong. For example, it has long been assumed that the best way to learn something is to sit down, preferably in a straight-backed chair, with no music or television noise in the background, read about a subject, then do multiple exercises to be sure you have learned the material.

Some students probably can learn this way. But in reality, this is probably the *least* effective way for people with ADD to learn. Though the minds of people with ADD are every bit as good as the minds of people who do not have ADD, their methods of arriving at conclusions, and sometimes the conclusions themselves, are different.

Because ADD is considered to be a *disorder*, a tendency exists to think of the ADD way as wrong or impaired. For people with ADD, that is a deadly assumption. It cuts off many options and perpetuates the concept that there is only one right way of doing things. In communication, when conversations are limited in this way, the non-ADD speaker tends to talk down to the person with ADD or discounts what could be valuable input. Unfortunately, the person with ADD often supports this contention, thinking he *should* be more like the non-ADD person and stifling his natural responses.

Consider Thomas, a gifted engineer. He is inventive and can solve any mechanical problem brought to his attention. In meetings, though, he tends to remain very quiet. Because he is afraid to let his coworkers know how he arrives at his solutions, he doesn't speak up. He just does the job when needed.

Thomas learned to operate like this long ago, because people who were wired differently criticized his way of doing things. He learned that they assumed his way was *wrong* because it wasn't the way recommended in the textbooks. Fortunately, Thomas never gave his way up, but think of the benefits to his coworkers if he had spoken up in work meetings and explained his viewpoint and methodology.

The Uh-Huh Phenomenon

As we have said, people who do not have ADD usually assume that the people they speak to actually listen to them. That assumption gets reinforced when the listeners says "uh-huh" during the conversation. When they hear that, speakers assume that the listeners are agreeing with a point they have made.

People with ADD, however, might just say "uh-huh" automatically. If you do this while someone is talking to you, you are leading that person to believe you are listening to them. In reality, you might not be listening well enough to recall what is being said even a short time later or to translate any agreements you inadvertently made into action. For example, consider Karen.

"Karen, will you bring the final figures on the Jacobson report to the meeting at two o'clock?" her supervisor asks.

Karen answers, "Uh-huh."

Two o'clock rolls around, and Karen arrives at the meeting, but she is empty handed.

"Where are the figures I asked for?" her irate colleague asks

"What figures?" Karen asks.

Was Karen lying when she agreed to bring the figures to the meeting? Why did she agree to something she wasn't going to do? Pretty soon, the feeling around the office is that you can't count on Karen. She's irresponsible. She's undisciplined. And if this type of behavior happens too often, Karen's job could be in jeopardy.

The Uh-huh Phenomenon has struck again.

As someone with ADD, you may often appear to be listening and say "uh-huh" not because you are lying but because you superficially hear someone saying something to you. Being a people pleaser, you nod and say "uh-huh" as if you took in the message. If asked at that very moment, you might be able to repeat the request, but moments later, it will have left you because you did not perceive it at a deep enough level to really hear it.

A deeper level of recognition is necessary before your "uh-huh" would mean that you agree to do whatever is in question. The sender of the message, however, cannot tell the difference between uh-huh, I hear you, and uh-huh, I agree to do what you've just asked. Worse yet, you probably don't realize whether you did or did not actually commit to something. Your automatic "uh-huh" response lies outside your conscious awareness.

To turn an agreement into actual action takes a third stage of commitment, which requires a still deeper level of information assimilation. That level of thought is not usually tapped when a person with ADD says, "uh-huh." For work partners to deal with this, the speaker must ask directly for affirmation. It's best, of course, if that request is made nicely, which shouldn't be too hard if you realize that the person with ADD sincerely needs your help.

For example, you could say to Karen, "Did you hear what I said?" Then wait for a response other than "uh-huh." I'd strongly recommend making eye contact at this stage. You might say, while touching Karen's hand, "Thanks so much. I appreciate your bringing the report to the two o'clock meeting." You've restated the request in a gracious way and, by touching Karen's hand, have focused her attention on you and raised her level of consciousness so she can hear you better.

If you are the person with ADD, it's a good idea to talk with your coworkers and explain this situation to them. I tell people, "Please be sure I've really heard what you want, because I don't want to let you down." Most people really appreciate this and are willing to help. Once in a while, someone considers it dependency and doesn't want to assist. That's their choice—but it is not dependency. This has to do with the chemistry of the brain that responds verbally without full knowledge of what is being responded to and what is to be done about it.

Speaking Impulsively

Many people who do not have ADD assume that a thought process precedes a response. For people with ADD, that does not necessarily happen. Impulsivity is often a problem for people with ADD. Though many people who have ADD have learned to laugh at their verbal impulsivity, it is really no laughing matter. Many, many things come out of their mouths unexpectedly, and they are often as surprised as listeners.

Imagine agreeing to take on a large project just because someone asked for volunteers, when you know you are already swamped. Perhaps motivated by the desire to be a nice guy, or maybe because of the exciting sound of the project, you volunteered before you gave it any thought. Backing out after you've volunteered would be tough indeed, especially after your coworkers thank you and discuss how glad they are to have you take on the project.

When you find yourself in a predicament like this, there is one—and only one—way to get out of it: confess, and the sooner the better, unless you can figure out some way to actually get the work done and stay alive in the process.

This type of speaking before you think can also damage interpersonal relationships. Suppose your auto body shop partner proudly shows you the car he just painted and asks, "How do you like this new paint color I mixed?" You respond, "Yuck. It stinks." Sure, to your eye it looks awful, but think about it: your partner would not have mixed a color he thought looked awful and then be proud of it. Oh, how you wish you'd kept your mouth shut!

In working with your impulsivity *before* it causes trouble for you, remember that your sensitivity is probably driving what comes out of your mouth. Though you might speak without thinking first, you do not speak without feeling first. Your job is to become aware of what you're feeling.

Think about the last time or two you put your foot in your mouth. What were you really feeling? Be honest.

Remember when your boss asked you to turn in that budget by 5 p.m., and you immediately answered, "Get real!" Maybe you were feeling overwhelmed. You wanted to push away that feeling of inadequacy, and "Get real!" is what popped out—at your boss, no less.

Once you've established what causes your anxiety, your vulnerable points, talk to yourself. Say, I am adequate. I have power. I am valuable. I'll accept me no matter what. I did the best I could. By nurturing that part of you that you previously may have been rejecting, you lay the groundwork for being less defensive. You can do it.

If your impulsivity still gets the best of you on occasion, all you can do is be honest and say, "I'm sorry. I wish I'd kept my mouth shut."

Speaking the Truth

People pleasing is a major problem for people with ADD. The reason behind it is quite understandable: having been told that the way you do things is wrong or noticing that the way you do things is often different from others, you may have grown to feel very inadequate and unacceptable. It's only natural to want to see yourself as adequate and acceptable, but from those desires a very bad habit can develop: lying.

Bosses, supervisors, or anyone else in a position of authority are especially likely to be the recipients of this behavior. The person with ADD might tell her boss what she thinks he wants to hear, although, that might be exactly the opposite from the way things really are.

Consider Candice. Candice is not a pathological liar. In fact, she usually doesn't even tell white lies. Here's how she tells her story:

"All I ever wanted to be was a nurse. Nursing school was really hard for me, but I finally made it through and passed the licensing exam. I started out working in ICU at a busy hospital and loved it, but the hours were unpredictable, and I had to quit when I started a family. Now I work in a small clinic. It's not nearly as exciting as ICU. And I'm in trouble a lot because I can never get my reports in on time. I'm even worried about getting fired.

"Yesterday, when my supervisor asked me about the summaries due months ago, I told her I'd left them at home and would bring them in tomorrow. But the truth is, I haven't even started them. I wish I was back in the emergency room. We were so busy that no one expected us to keep up with our notes."

Hypersensitive to criticism, Candice fears failure and needs approval. In hope of getting that approval, she lied to her supervisor.

What she did not say to her supervisor was that she had no idea how to keep track of all the information she was expected to put in the patients' charts. She did not know how to organize the writing of the reports. Furthermore, she could not sit still long enough to try to figure out how to do it.

However, she did want to keep that particular job so that she would have regular hours and be able to spend time with her child. She wanted to be a good employee.

Candice's boss has no way of knowing what the real truth is, because Candice tells her boss what she thinks the boss wants to hear. This robs her supervisor of the opportunity to help her. Both Candice and her boss lose out in this situation, and it is very possible that Candice will lose her job.

What could Candice have done? Ideally, she would have told her boss about her limitations at the outset and asked for help in organizing her work. Her boss might have suggested putting Candice on a schedule from the very start, having her make regular short-term reports. A computer-drafted report outline would not have been hard to develop and could be filled in with individual patient details.

Setting aside some time on a weekly or monthly basis to allow for in-office report writing would help many employees who would otherwise become overwhelmed when a lot of reports were to accumulate.

Occasionally there is a boss who does not want to make these kinds of accommodations. Usually, though, if you approach the person with simple, clear communication about your needs, a boss or supervisor would be happy to help. Don't expect your boss to design a program to meet your needs, though. You be the one to suggest what you need—and be specific. Talk in a friendly way, saying, "Such-and-such is what will help me do the kind of job you want me to do, and the kind of job I am capable of doing. Thank you for helping me."

In Candice's case, because she did not start out following this kind of plan, all she can do is confess and then present some suggestions. The worst thing she could do would be to continue to ignore the problem or try to fix it on her own. Many supervisors appreciate an employee who recognizes having made a mistake, even a big one, and who is willing to fix it so it isn't repeated. It is worth an honest try.

"Everyone Else Knows More than I Do"

Because people with ADD often have had many experiences with failure, they may begin to assume that they will always be wrong and everyone else will always be right. That assumption influences the way in which they communicate with people.

The message has constantly been communicated to you that there is something wrong with you. How, then, could you be expected to believe in yourself, your views, and your opinions? Even when you arrive at acceptable answers, you are likely to have arrived at them in a different way from than of your non-ADD counterparts. Remember all the times that your schoolwork was marked wrong because the process you used to get to an answer was different?

The situation becomes even more complicated when you use intuition to arrive at your solutions. You "just feel what to do in your gut," or you simply have a sense that such-and-such is wrong with the person, machine, or drawing. Later you confirm that sense by going through generally agreed-upon steps to "prove" your position. But the reality may be that you knew the correct answer using your intuition. And you also secretly know that that intuition is very seldom, if ever, wrong.

However, even you may question your intuitive skills. Do you dare to share your unconventional approach with your well-trained, educated colleagues or teammates? If you don't, you run the risk of not getting feedback that will reinforce your way of doing things. Alone, you are likely to discount your skill.

You do have a need to communicate with like-minded people, but you may or may not find them in your workplace or business. You might have to rely on others who share your learning style and are further down the road of experience.

I know how hard it is to communicate thoughts and ideas in the workplace when you hold an opinion that differs from that of your colleagues.

For example, in my counseling years, I recall the day I leaned back in my chair with my eyes closed, wondering what could be keeping the man in front of me from overcoming his depression, which was yielding to neither counseling nor drug therapy. A light bulb went off in my head, so to speak, and in my mind I saw a school-age child who was restless, painfully trapped in a school desk. I visualized him daydreaming and intuitively felt that this man had ADD.

Immediately my rational mind countered, "But it's supposed to go away at puberty." Fortunately, I pursued my *intuition*, exploring other situations methodically, and found, to my surprise and delight, that my client was not the only man who suffered from improper diagnosis. Now, thankfully, many people are being helped who previously remained incompletely or improperly treated.

I promise you I was told many times that I was wrong. Thank goodness I was provided the courage to believe in myself and my convictions.

Great difficulties can occur, however, when you try to use your intuitive sense and communicate that sense to a coworker or client who is not very empathetic. You may want to ask yourself, "Do I sometimes, or even often, find myself backing down from my opinion because someone else has a differing view?" Whether we are talking about automobile engines, hairstyles, or the best stocks and bonds, you will have your reasons for why you believe as you do. Do not automatically assume that the other guy is right and you are wrong.

Sure, recheck your facts and get all the information together that you need to support your view. I'm not suggesting that you go on intuition alone. Remember, you have a good head on your shoulders. Use it. And don't be afraid to communicate what you know and what you've learned.

Everything Is Either Black or White

Part of what I call the on-off switch influences the tendency in people with ADD to feel, think, and act in extremes. This switch is a neurobiochemical mechanism. It seems to make people be either very active or very inactive, or very happy or very sad, or see things as all right or all wrong. Consequently, people with ADD tend to see situations as having two possible outcomes, one on either extreme, and no options in the middle of the spectrum. A winner or a loser—those are the only choices.

This on-off view also applies to communication. If a person with ADD isn't comfortable with what his coworker is saying in a particular conversation, he might automatically discount everything else that person says or does. The person with ADD would probably not initiate a dialogue to try to discover why differences exist or what they are about. Without that communication, there's no chance to reconcile those differences. There is no opportunity for negotiation. Chances are, everyone loses.

Rarely do two people see things in exactly the same way. This is as true in the workplace as it is in any other part of your life. Communication in general, and dialogue in particular, is the key to moving forward to accomplish the goals of any job. Anyone who has tried to work with someone who routinely sees only one side of an issue knows how frustrating that can be.

Let's look at Hank's situation. Hank has some office furniture to sell. He's moving into smaller quarters and has to get rid of it quickly. Besides, he needs the money. He does find a buyer, but that person cannot pay for the furniture all at one time. Hank agrees to four equal payments. He collects the first payment and lets the man take the furniture. When some time has gone by and Hank has not received another payment, he calls the buyer. The buyer apologizes and says he'll send a payment the next day. However, Hank receives only half of the amount they had agreed on. More time goes by with no further response.

One day, Hank decides he has had enough. He decides to go to the man's place of business and take back the furniture right then. When he arrives, he's primed to press his demand. To Hank's surprise, the man asks whether he'll leave the furniture if he pays Hank in full. Hank barely knows how to respond because that was not one of the options he'd thought about.

Hank recovers his composure and accepts the cash—and he learned a lesson. If two people can talk about the issues rather than fight over the differences, they can arrive at arrangements that are beneficial to both of them.

"But I Said . . . "

Many people with ADD make the false assumption that if they are talking, they are communicating. That assumption just isn't true.

For example, consider a compulsive talker who barely takes a breath between sentences, leaving no room for questions, much less comments. There's little communication going on in such a situation. Usually the listener is so overwhelmed with information that much of what is being said is lost. What's left is likely to be pushed away in self-defense.

If you have a tendency toward compulsive talking, you probably have Highly Structured ADD. You are not "bad" because of your style, but you need to realize that much of what you say is probably going to be lost.

There are several reasons why you have this tendency to talk compulsively. Part of it is just your body chemistry, which steers you to the path of compulsive speech without the ability to talk and listen in short segments. Your mind, no doubt, has many tracks running at once, and the results of all those thoughts just pour out of your mouth.

Then, too, your eagerness to be heard contributes to trying to get everything said—and said fast. You are so clearly focused on yourself that you forget to check on what the other person is hearing. You forget, too, that you may need to modify what you are saying based on what the other person needs or wants—the give and take that makes real dialogue.

Breaking the habit of compulsive talking takes practice. Here's one way to work with it. Before you begin talking, make a mental outline— or even an outline on paper, if you feel that is necessary—of what you want to cover. Then divide the whole outline into segments, short ones that allow for breaks in your talking. Next, practice talking about only one segment at a time. Then stop. If necessary, take notes on the other person's response.

This may seem drastic, but it might be what's needed at first to help you meet your goal: focusing your attention on what that other person is saying. You might even want to wear a vibrating timer in your pocket for a while to help train yourself to take breaks. You *can* train yourself—and there's no time like the present.

Don't We All Think Alike?

Strange as it may seem, many people with ADD assume that everyone can understand and appreciate how they think and are purposely discounting what they are saying. The speaker who has ADD never considers the possibility that the listener may not be able to understand what the person with ADD is saying.

Because the person who has ADD has not fit into the system for so long, the assumption may be made that this person is automatically wrong and the person without ADD is automatically right. That is just not a valid assumption. The reality is that many creative people with ADD think "head and shoulders" above their colleagues. Visionaries who are ahead of their time, inventors who see the future, and creative people of all kinds often get ideas and develop skills years before the public is ready for their offerings. And many of these people have ADD.

You can test the hypothesis that you are ahead of others in your thinking by breaking one of your thoughts down into smaller parts. For example, suppose you've designed a shopping mall that has a food court in the middle. The only problem is that the year is 1930, and shopping is done in downtown department stores.

When someone ignores your suggestions or discounts what you've done, you might ask, "Have you ever thought how useful it might be not to have to go so far from home to do your shopping?"

Watch the person's face and see whether there is some sparkle of interest or hint that they see the connection to your shopping mall concept. If not, you probably have gone over his head. You'll have to decide whether you want to talk with this person more on his level so that you don't overwhelm him. Those people who have functioned on a more mundane, or noncreative, level most of their lives may feel threatened, or at least uncomfortable, with too much newness all at once. Communication will be aided by slowing down and giving small bits of new information at a time.

The enthusiasm that many people with ADD have may be lost on someone who does not think or behave the same way. Therefore, when you rush up to a coworker to communicate a suggestion or proposal that is important to you, you may find you are less welcome than you would like. And talking a mile a minute does not mean you can make the other person catch up with you.

As a result, it's possible you will be ignored, discounted, told why your proposal won't work. What sometimes has happened in situations like this, is that the person with ADD has communicated more of his emotions than the specific content of his proposal. Feeling so good and excited, you might have substituted emotion for accuracy of information.

For people who analyze or think more than they feel, you may simply find you are on a different communication channel. Since you are the one trying to initiate the communication, you will need to change how you present yourself.

Imagine that you have just landed a huge sales deal. You even did a great job of tying up loose ends, taking into account many details you might normally have missed. You feel so proud of yourself and excited about your accomplishment that you want to share it immediately with a coworker.

So you rush up to the nearest person, a research supervisor in the adjoining department, and excitedly share the results of your meeting. She looks at you rather suspiciously and says, "Well, a lot of things could go wrong with that kind of deal. What are you going to do if ... ?" After delivering a short list of possible problems, she turns back to the work on her desk as if dismissing you and your victory. Feeling devastated, you walk slowly away, wondering why other people can't appreciate you.

What your coworker said might have been true. With almost any deal, there are things that could go wrong, and you are indeed capable of thinking through those possibilities and coming up with contingency plans. The problem with the conversation was that you were communicating on two different levels. You were communicating your emotions about the deal and your sense of accomplishment. She was communicating her factual analysis of the elements of the deal. Neither of you was right or wrong, but your communication was doomed because you were coming from different planes of thought.

Next time, choose the person to share with more carefully. Then say what you want to say, something like, "I'm really proud of myself, and I want to share how I feel with someone who can help me celebrate."

Putting It in Writing

Written business communication can be a major problem for people with ADD. For many people with ADD, writing is a dreaded chore, and just getting around to doing what feels like a chore creates stress. I'll do it in a minute, you say to yourself. However, that minute is likely never to come. Even if it does, the information that was to be committed to paper has vanished.

Part of your problem with writing might be that the creative spontaneity that drove you to focus on your idea is gone now that you need to take that idea and write it down. Unaided by that creativity, your mind is likely to drift, which makes writing very difficult. After all, when you write something down, you're restating ground you've already been over in your mind. That tends to be boring for people with ADD, and if a chore is boring, there's a good chance it will never be done.

The trick is to keep your written comments short. If you do have to write a more lengthy report, divide it into segments. Otherwise, don't think about what you're doing as writing: think of it as taking notes. Your mind-set will help you get to the task and complete it. Then reward yourself for a job finished.

Documentation—whether it's keeping track of your mileage to and from a meeting, notes on a medical patient, or notes on a sales meeting—is often the bane of a talented person's existence. What must be kept in mind is this: do it now, this instant, or it won't get done. If you tackle it now, it may be difficult. If you put it off until it becomes just one item in a list of chores that were never completed, the situation becomes overwhelming and sometimes impossible.

Some people like to keep a small tape recorder in their pocket or purse to record their assessments of conversations. If you do carry a tape recorder, record your thoughts immediately—even while the other person is still there with you. Later a secretary can write down what you've recorded. This is much, much easier than driving back to your office after the meeting, trying to remember what was said, and staring at a blank piece of paper that is supposed to be filled with your summary of the meeting.

Learn to make outlines and write only in outline form. Pick the main headings or topics and limit the number of words you write. You can go back afterward to see whether you said enough to convey the information appropriately. Remember, you do not need to justify how you came to your conclusions. You don't need to write lengthy stories to support your summary or plan. Just get to the point and stick to it.

Actually, You're Ahead of the Game

Many people with ADD are very communicative, both verbally and in writing. Consider the number of entertainers, deejays, talk show hosts, speakers, and preachers who make their living through verbal communication. If you have these skills naturally, speaking in front of others might come easily to you, and it might be something you love to do.

Part of the inherent ability you have with language comes from the fact that you process things simultaneously on multiple levels, so you have endless material to draw upon. This is the same skill used by the stand-up comic; what happened on the way to the podium becomes fodder for talk.

People with the ability to think on their feet and translate those thoughts quickly into speech do not *write* speeches. Rather, extemporaneous speaking is the form the communication takes. This is akin to the music played by free jazz musicians, an improvised style in which the instruments "talk" back and forth to each other, in contrast to that played in traditional concert halls. Neither is better or worse: they are just very different.

As I mentioned earlier, for me this ability to think on so many levels at once, an ability that results from my ADD, is the skill that enabled me to become a successful radio talk show host and professional speaker. If you have ADD and you love to speak extemporaneously, communicating your thoughts to a large number of people at once, there are many careers in which that skill can be put to good use.

You might not realize it, but many people who do not have ADD (and some who do, especially those with Highly Structured ADD) are terrified at the prospect of getting up in front of other people and speaking. If you are comfortable speaking in front of others, and even thrive on it like I do, you have been blessed with a very valuable skill, and you are way ahead of the game in the workplace.

Improving Communication: How Do You Rate?

If communication is not one of your strengths right now, don't worry. You can learn to become an effective communicator.

The first thing you need to do is determine the function of the communication you're considering. Ask yourself these questions:

- What kind of communication is called for?

- Does this situation require just talking to people, i.e., one-way communication?

- Would it be more appropriate to have a dialogue, a communication give-and-take, so that you come out of the conversation with more information than you had going in?

- Is the goal to try to solve a particular problem, working with a group of people?

- Is the person receiving your communication a better listener or a better reader?

Once you're clear about the function of the communication, then you can decide whether written or verbal communication will best lead to the outcome you desire. Finally, you need to plan how much time you will need for the communication and when you want to do it.

Do a little thinking about these categories now, before you need to use them at work. You might want to write them down, so you can become more familiar with them. Before you know it, they will become automatic.

Now let's see how you would rate the communication you've had in the recent past. Make a list of the last five communications you have had, and label them according to the types listed above. Rate each of them as either "great," "okay," or "needs improvement." If you're not sure how to rate yourself, consider these questions: Did you talk too much? How well did you listen? Were you able to get your point across? Did you learn anything from the other person? Were you comfortable?

Don't worry if you realize that you need improvement—that's the first step in building your communication strengths.

Learning to Say "No"

One of the most important words you can learn to use when you are communicating in the workplace is *no*. That's because taking on too much work—so that you don't really get anything done well, or done at all—is a major error made by many people with ADD. Although part of your motivation in taking on such a heavy workload may be to help yourself focus by applying pressure, the end result may be to acquire more than you or anyone else could possibly accomplish. That can lead to serious consequences: a bad reputation, loss of status, a label of irresponsibility, and possibly loss of job opportunities or even loss of the job itself.

You may be afraid to say no for fear of displeasing someone, but you need to know that you will actually gain people's respect if you set realistic limits on what you can and cannot do. There are ways you can say no to someone asking you to take on extra assignments and still help that person get the work done. Think of ways you can get some of the work done for him yourself, or try to come up with a solution that does not involve you but still meets his needs.

For example, your coworker may have asked you to help with a project due tomorrow. However, you have your own project due, and that work would be jeopardized if you took any time away from your project. You don't have to respond to the request with a flat-out no. Instead, you might ask, "What needs to be done?"

When you get the answer, you might realize that a worker down the hall has just the skills needed, as well as some slack time, and might be willing to help. You might say, "I'll finish my project and if I have any time, I'll be glad to help you out. But, why don't you check around to see if someone else is available in case I don't get finished on time." You might add, "Go ahead and ask me next time, though, because I'd be happy to help you if I weren't on deadline, too."

Those of us with ADD are often effusive and creative and don't easily see boundaries. In fact, it's exactly because we don't see artificial boundaries that we are so creative. That can also sidetrack us. It's important to set limits on ourselves, so we can stay goal oriented when that is necessary. Part of our asset is also our liability, since every moment contains new opportunities. However, in order to stay with our creative projects to completion, we must set priorities and be able to say no to the myriad other opportunities that we see.

Talking Your Way through Assignments

Many people with ADD learned to talk their way through school. Though feeling guilty about having done this, it was actually a useful tool to deal with learning situations that didn't fit. Similarly when you are confronted on the job with an assignment that doesn't fit very well, you may be able to talk your way through it.

It's important to guard against deluding yourself, though. If you are in a situation that requires technical information or skill, it is not a good idea to try to fake your way through it. But let's say you are selling a carload of "as is" merchandise. The consumer is then being made aware to use his own judgment, and you are not trying to convince anyone of something you know nothing about.

The gift of gab is a useful tool that can be polished to a high level of brilliance. If you have Outwardly Expressive ADD and are talkative by nature, enjoy refining that gift. Just be selective in how and where you use your skills.

"The Way I See It, . . . "

Communication in the workplace can break down when two people with differing opinions discuss their ideas, but it doesn't have to be that way. You can become an effective force for solving those problems if you learn to voice your opinions with confidence but realize that you don't have to argue. Instead of arguing, try stating the following fact: "I see things differently from you."

You also don't have to convince anyone that you are right and they are wrong. Neither do you need to drop your way of seeing things because the other person has a different perspective. Even if you are talking to an authority, remember that this person is assessing the world through his or her own brain wiring, and you are seeing things through yours. That does not automatically make either of you right or wrong.

I've noticed at national ADD conferences that the many professionals attending have a variety of opinions and ways to deal with ADD. This is because we all share what we know best. We really can't completely get into another person's skin to feel and see the world as that person does, so we develop ways to work with ADD, or anything else, based on what we've found works best with ourselves. We can make educated guesses about others who are not too different from us, but the final judgment about what will work for you must be left up to you.

So, speak up and say what you think. Be confident. Remember, you don't have to put the other person down to prove that your way is right. Just say, "Thanks for trying to help me and offering your opinion. I'll think about it. I'll check out your way and then see what works best for me."

Communication without Words

There is no doubting the strength of verbal communication in making contact with, and doing business with, other people. But you might not have realized that nonverbal communication may be even more powerful. Nonverbal communication is more likely to put you ill at ease than someone's words, and the hypersensitivity of people with ADD means you are more likely than the average person to notice it.

Nonverbal communication includes the body positions of the speaker, tone of voice, and facial expressions. Rolling eyes, smirks, folded arms, and turning the body away from the speaker are a few common forms of nonverbal communication. These actions are driven by the speaker's internal feelings and may be telling truths that aren't being verbalized.

Haven't you had someone come up to you saying, "I'm so glad to see you, buddy. What a guy you are,"—only to feel that he doesn't even remember your name as he looks away to someone else who is passing. Have you ever asked someone with a downturned mouth, tense facial muscles, and a vertical crease in his forehead, "How are you?" only to be answered, "Fine." You know by looking at him that that person is not fine, but what you can't tell is whether he is simply unaware of how he's feeling, doesn't want to talk about it, or doesn't want you to notice.

Conversely, I've known people doing business who always keep a straight face, not changing their expressions even when you present a completed project that absolutely delights them. They do not communicate nonverbally. This type of person is very easy to misread, especially for people with ADD who tend to think the worst because of their own feelings of inadequacy.

Silence is also communication. For example, you might have an idea at work that is so far ahead of its time that others don't understand it. You may read their silence, however, as meaning they don't like the idea. Be sure to ask, "What do you think?" I know that is a scary question sometimes when you feel insecure inside, but it's better to ask the question than make an inaccurate assumption.

Many people with ADD have also learned to "fake it," using nonverbal communication to cover their true feelings. Though facial expressions are usually not planned, they may be, so you need to get to know a person to know what they mean by what they do. Also, remember that not every nonverbal behavior means the same thing every time it's used. I find that I cross my arms in front of my body when I'm cold. This has nothing to do with standing my ground, a frequent misinterpretation of that body position.

In many ways, people with ADD are at a distinct advantage when it comes to reading the meanings behind nonverbal communication. Not only are they sensitive to this form of communication, but they can often see the most subtle cues imaginable.

For example, the slightest inflection, backing away, or shift in stance tells Tom, a salesman, that he's losing a sale and had better change the direction he's going with his sales pitch. Consider Jenny, a counselor who seems to know what her client is feeling before any words are spoken. She is able to adjust her therapeutic interventions to fit her client's needs due to her sensitivity to what she is perceiving nonverbally. This helps her client get in touch with her true feelings and saves a lot of talking time. Tom and Jenny's sensitivity to nonverbal cues has helped them become highly effective in their careers.

However, reading someone's nonverbal communication and comparing it to his verbal signals can also lead to confusion, because mixed messages create havoc. When someone calls you on a nonverbal expression, you need to be honest, if at all possible. At least acknowledge that you have some feelings other than those you are verbally discussing, and honestly say you would rather not share them at that time. If they are not in the best interest of the listener, you may need to say, "I'm working on how I feel." If they have nothing to do with the person, you need to say so. If they are positive, say something like, "I was just thinking about how we can go about marketing your idea. My frown was about some problems I see that I'm sure we can overcome. It wasn't because of your idea: I think it's great."

On the other hand, people with ADD may have trouble inhibiting their nonverbal communication. One doctor I know, a highly skilled, excellent professional whose ADD characteristics include some anxiety and compulsive behaviors, discovered he was frightening his patients with his frowns and grimaces. Granted, he was a worrier, constantly worrying about every little thing that could go wrong, but it was not appropriate for him to convey every one of those worries to his patients.

In situations where a straight face is an asset, the nonverbal expressiveness of a person with ADD, especially someone who has Outwardly Expressive ADD, may show enthusiasm during a negotiation when no communication would have been preferable.

By heightening your awareness to the particular expressions you have, you can begin to censor your expressions. This will give you control in situations where you need it. Consider asking a friend to help you. None of us is really aware of the gestures we make unconsciously, at least not until our attention is called to them.

Typical gestures you may have to contend with could be rolling your eyes, throwing your hands up in the air, huffing and puffing, raising an eyebrow, or giving a look of disdain. Learning to mask them when you choose takes into consideration the real world in which you work. This is not just people pleasing. Rather, you are quite aware of what you are doing and are acting purposefully to keep your feelings more to yourself.

For example, let's say you feel your boss is inept. The bottom line is that she has power over you and your job and, if she chooses, can relieve you of the latter or otherwise make your life quite difficult. You don't need that, so just acknowledge to yourself what you really feel, which feelings you are going to express, and which feelings you would do better to keep to yourself. If the situation is too bad, begin to look around for another job opportunity. Meanwhile, you will be gaining mastery over your nonverbal communications.

Almost everyone could use some improvement in their communication skills, whether nonverbal or verbal. If you are ADD, just realize that your stronger and weaker areas will probably be different than those of your non-ADD counterparts. Still, all of us need to communicate. When you improve communication skills in the workplace, you will enjoy the benefits of improved relationships with your coworkers, improved productivity, and greater self-esteem.

5

Interpersonal Relationships on the Job

M ore jobs are probably gained and lost because of interpersonal issues than for any other reason. In this chapter I will help you learn how to be successful in relationships with the people in your workplace. Even if you have opted for self-employment rather than working for someone else, the relationships you build with coworkers, customers, and suppliers can make or break your business.

Besides how to build trusting relationships with your boss and coworkers, we'll discuss the pros and cons of telling them about your ADD, as well as how to do it. We'll also talk about office politics and guidelines for working on a team, a crucial set of skills that will make your life more pleasant and effective. And, yes, we'll talk about office romance.

ADD Is Not an Excuse

How do you know whether or not you are using your ADD as an excuse? Check your feelings. It is perfectly normal to need to feel adequate and to want to feel strong, secure, and skillful. All of these factors lead to feelings of self-worth.

If you are feeling inadequate, helpless, or lacking in some way, you need something that will make you feel protected and more powerful to get what you want. As you search for that "something," you are likely to recall all the times you felt inadequate. Because many of them resulted from your having ADD, you are likely to blame your current feelings on that. Although your ADD may be the reason why you are having problems, using ADD as an excuse rather than an explanation will only cause others to discount you or become irritated with you.

The difference between an excuse and an explanation lies in your motive. If you are simply complaining, helplessly giving in to the reason for why you are having difficulty, you are using your ADD as an excuse. Others will feel it. Everyone has problems and feelings of inadequacy, and no one wants to be reminded of them nor feel he has have to take care of someone who has given in to the very feelings he is trying to avoid.

Your key to success is your understanding and taking responsibility to do something about your ADD. If you are actively working with your ADD to make changes in your work habits that will help you to become successful, then chances are you are simply using your ADD to explain your behavior or difficulty in a specific situation. If you are actively working to help yourself, others may want to help you, also. Consequently, as you give information and request assistance from your co-workers, you are likely to discover exactly the support you desire.

Ultimately, though, it is your responsibility to provide what you need. Others only help voluntarily. Respect them for this.

All healthy relationships are based on mutual respect, but how can you hope to receive respect from someone if you don't feel deserving? Self-respect must come first. Rather than beat up on yourself or express critical judgments about your inadequacies, you must come to an understanding of ADD's impact on your life and take responsibility to counteract its influence. You will be acting in a perfectly responsible manner if you ask for (not demand) specific help because you have ADD. You can tell another person the warning signs that your ADD has kicked in and give that person permission to bring your attention to it.

Simple honesty about your way of doing things sets the scene for you to receive the acknowledgment you desire as someone who is self-responsible. Others will be able to trust you because you will trust yourself to be responsible. It's that easy.

Consider Sylvester. Sylvester's job required him to keep track of the inventory of supplies needed in the welding shop where he worked. When he was first hired, he nodded that he understood what was expected of him. The shop manager assumed Sylvester had his job under control. You can imagine his surprise when materials ran out.

When asked what happened, Sylvester blandly said, "I have ADD. I can't help it." Needless to say, his boss was not happy with him.

By not explaining his ADD in the first place, so his boss could understand the ways it affected him, Sylvester failed to take responsibility for it. Neither did he ask for a reminder from a coworker. Instead Sylvester's ADD became an excuse for his failure. To a great degree, Sylvester's problem was not his ADD: the problem was his failure to take responsibility for his situation and make the necessary accommodations.

When his boss continued to question him, Sylvester demonstrated the feelings of helplessness that often accompanies ADD.

"There's nothing I can do about it," he said. "I'm just dumb."

Sylvester didn't expect anything more than failure for himself. He accepted this job with the assumption that he wouldn't be able to keep it very long, because he always "screwed things up." Low self-esteem presented much more of a problem for Sylvester than ADD ever would. He had received no training either growing up or as an adult as to how to manage his ADD. Consequently, he had no skills to deal with his ADD effectively. Nevertheless, as an adult in the workplace, it had become his responsibility to get the skills he needed.

His boss felt Sylvester had let him down, and he felt he could no longer trust Sylvester. Even after this incident, though, if Sylvester had been able to give his boss information about ADD, he might have rebuilt trust between the two of them. They could have worked out a plan so Sylvester wouldn't jeopardize himself or his coworkers. If he did that, his boss would have felt that Sylvester was acting responsibly, rather than just doing a sloppy job.

You must pay attention to the ways you are affected by your ADD. Then it becomes your responsibility to communicate to your coworkers how they can best work with you. You do not necessarily have to explain that you have ADD—or you can—but you must let others know what accommodations you need. And you can also ask them what they need.

You must learn to get along with people and respect their need for information. You have no choice if you want them to consider you fairly. Showing them that same respect will also improve your relationships with them.

The fact that you have ADD does not mean that you are to be excused from the normal requirements of a job. You have to be able to do the job with the help of *reasonable accommodation*, and you must take responsibility for discovering what that accommodation is. (See Appendix for more information about reasonable accommodation under the Americans with Disabilities Act.)

To Tell or Not to Tell

Should I tell my boss or coworkers about my ADD?

Before you can answer that question, I suggest that you ask yourself three other questions. First, Do I think this person will be able to benefit from the information I am sharing? Second, What do I want to get by sharing that information with this person? Third, Am I prepared to let the person know what accommodations I need?

When you have answered these three questions, you will either be in good shape to share the information about your ADD—or you will have decided not to. If you can clearly see that there will be a benefit to your sharing the information, and if you are willing to make suggestions to your boss or coworkers about how they might help you work more successfully, then it is probably a good idea to go ahead and discuss your ADD.

The key is that you must be willing to take responsibility for helping your boss or coworkers work more successfully with you. If you just want to tell them about your ADD so they can feel sorry for you, or because you want them to feel badly about having criticized you in a particular situation, then you will probably not be improving your workplace situation by discussing your ADD.

Suppose you have thought things through and decided that there would be some benefit in discussing your ADD. How can you tell whether your particular boss is open to hearing about your ADD? Here are some behaviors to watch out for, red flags that might indicate he or she might be unaccepting of differences:

- Being judgmental about *any* differences: "Henry knows the right way to stack boxes. Peter ought to have his head examined for the way he's going about the job."

- Labeling people or their behavior in negative ways if they do things differently from the boss. "Did you see the way that *foreigner* draws plans? She doesn't know a thing."

- Refusing to acknowledge that some inadequacies are beyond the control of the person: "She could do it if she just tried."

- Being so tied to production that people don't count: "I don't care what it takes to get the job done—your kids will have to wait."

- Blaming people for errors rather than trying to figure a better way to do things: "The fact that we missed this deadline was your fault. And don't tell me it's because we didn't have enough support staff: we don't need any more help. You're supposed to get this job done yourself."

- Appearing to be controlling and inflexible in his own life and with others: "I have to bring my car into the shop at exactly 9:15 this morning, and I don't care what you're doing right then."

How can you tell, on the other hand, that your boss would probably be open to accommodating your ADD and in fact would like to know how to help you become a more efficient employee? Notice whether your boss has some of the following behaviors or attitudes:

- He asks how you and your family are doing and waits to hear your answer.

- She helps other employees become more effective.

- He shares differences he has and asks for accommodation from employees.

- Appears emotionally flexible.

- She tries to offer solutions when someone makes a mistake or bumps into an obstacle, rather than placing blame.

If your boss generally seems to be an accommodating, flexible person, you might seriously want to consider sharing information about your ADD. I know many people for whom it would have been better to have shared that information, but didn't.

Consider Kenneth. As a floor salesman, Kenneth was a whiz. He knew all about his product and loved to talked to people about it. He just loved to sell, and, consequently, he was a great salesman, walking off with the top sales award every month. In fact, he did such a good job that management wanted to promote him to corporate sales, which would require him to sit at a desk all day and do his selling over the phone.

In order to assess how good the move would be for his career, Kenneth thought about how good the promotion would look on his resume and how proud the promotion would make him feel. Because he was flattered, Kenneth took the corporate job, bragging about his promotion. Unfortunately, Kenneth lasted only two months at his new job.

Although Kenneth's Outwardly Expressive ADD was an asset in selling on the floor, it proved to be an enormous liability for the desk job.

He couldn't sit at his desk for much more than ten minutes at a time, failed to complete paperwork, and talked too long with busy corporate officers. As a result, he was demoted back to floor sales.

Although that type of selling had been his forte, when Kenneth was demoted, he became depressed and no longer sold well. He was eventually fired when the little habits that were overlooked when he was a top salesman became too much of a nuisance. Suddenly his supervisor didn't like his being chronically five to ten minutes late to work, failing to do paperwork adequately, acting as a cutup on the floor, and talking at length to customers, although that previously had often led to increased sales.

Kenneth's real problem was that he just didn't know himself very well. If you have ADD, you must have a clear understanding of your abilities and know what works with those abilities and what doesn't. You must learn to respect those limits.

Career decisions based on thoughtfulness about whether and how to talk about ADD can then be wisely made. Know yourself, and those working with you will appreciate you whether you have ADD or not.

Office Politics

Listening with attention to the boss's boring stories, knowing when to go along with the crowd, and being seen at the right social functions are all aspects of office politics. Whether you like them or not, they not only exist but are an inevitable part of the routine in many workplaces.

The truth is that playing the game of office politics properly can mean the difference between success or failure on the job.

No one is exempt from office politics, but some people with ADD have a difficult time understanding the game, much less being able to play the game well. If you have Outwardly Expressive ADD, you probably do well in situations when the game of office politics includes socializing outside of work, especially in a party atmosphere. You're likely charismatic and well-liked, so socializing may be your cup of tea. You tend to be quick to pick up on others' moods, and if you like being helpful, you'll be right there for the other guy.

The problem for people with Outwardly Expressive ADD comes if they don't like the form the politics are taking. They tend to broadcast their dislike more loudly than might be wise. Impulsively exhibiting feelings that differ from the "powers that be," they can find themselves in hot water. Also, being expected to do something just because a superi-

or expects it may cause them to buck the system emphatically. To get along they'll have to be *very* valuable to the company despite going against the grain.

If your form of ADD tends to be more like the quieter, Inwardly Directed ADD, you may be off in dreamland rather than even being aware that the politics are going on. Often less openly interested in people than your Outwardly Expressive ADD counterparts, you may retreat into your area of expertise and hide from the politics. Unfortunately, though, office politics is just not something you can hide from. It's possible that if you withdraw into yourself without making social connections at your workplace, you might be passed over for promotions that your work itself deserves.

If you have Inwardly Directed ADD, you are probably very sensitive, and you may be more interested in the underdog than in the company powers. However, you are also likely to hide your feelings and simply end up feeling depressed. You may find outside interests away from work that seem to prevent you from participating in the politics, but job advancement may lag behind with this approach.

Even if you recognize the game of office politics for what it is and recognize the need to play the game, figuring out the strategy may not be easy. Based primarily on the needs of the people in power, each situation will be different, and there is no way to figure out one formula for what to do and when and how to do it. It can be very frustrating.

If you are Highly Structured ADD, you may actually do quite well playing office politics, especially if you are at all good at strategizing quickly. Using your sensitivity to advantage, taking a calculated approach to what you do socially, and strategically placing yourself in positions aligned with those in power, you could mastermind a scheme for playing that would win a prize.

You could also get into trouble if you perceive a situation differently from the people in charge. Because inflexibility tends to be one of the characteristics of people with Highly Structured ADD, you may clash with those in charge. That's no way to play politics—unless you choose to conspire against those in power and build your own system. And that certainly has its own dangers.

Either not picking up on the situation or purposely deciding not to get involved, some employees simply choose not to play the game of office politics. Whether you have ADD or not, that rarely works.

For example, consider Wilson. Wilson didn't "get it" when he was asked if he would buy cookies from his supervisor's daughter's club. He said, "No, thank you: I don't eat sweets." Not understanding that the request had nothing to do with whether Wilson ate sweets or not, he failed to do what his supervisor needed him to do: play the game of "let's all support the boss's daughter." Because of that simple misunderstanding, Wilson became characterized as uncooperative. The word around the business was that Wilson was not a team player. When promotions came around, Wilson was left out.

"Did You Hear About . . . ?"

Talking about people when they are not present has probably gone on as long as groups of people have gotten together to pass the time. Sometimes harmless and often not meant to be hurtful, gossip in the workplace undermines morale, wastes time, and reduces efficiency and productivity.

Though most people gossip now and again, chronic gossips live for the opportunity to pass on something new they have heard, seen, or suspected. Often without checking the truth in their bit of information, the gossip can quickly spread a rumor that has little or no substance. Gossiping is frequently a way for people to vent their feelings without having to confront a person or situation directly. However, that approach almost always makes the situation worse.

Especially if you have Highly Structured ADD, you may need to watch carefully that you don't become a habitual gossip. People with this type of ADD are prone to talking, so it's a natural avenue to use. Listen carefully to what you are talking about. Be sure you are not spending your time talking about people or problems that need direct action or negotiation instead of talk behind the scenes. If you have Outwardly Expressive ADD, you are probably less likely to be a chronic gossip, but you will still need to watch against speaking impulsively.

Gossip helps people who have low self-esteem feel more important. Can you picture yourself being the center of attention, with all eyes focused on you, while you share the latest juicy morsel of gossip? Because what you are saying seems to be important to a lot of people, you are likely to feel important as a result of telling it.

You deserve better. You can increase your feelings of importance more directly without falling into the trap of gossiping. For example, use your creativity to figure out a way to solve the difficulty that is being gossiped about, or draw upon your courage, going directly to the person being discussed and getting the straight story.

Simply say, "I heard that you dislike my project. I would like to know whether you see the situation differently. I'd like to know what it is you don't like, and perhaps I can modify it so we're both pleased."

The only time that getting involved in office gossip may be necessary is when your boss or supervisor gossips to you. At that point, your decision about whether to get involved should be based on whether you are asked a direct question. If you are asked a direct question, your best bet is usually to answer honestly but with tact. If you are not asked a direct question, it is probably better simply to listen without committing yourself one way or the other to what your boss is saying.

Remember that anyone who gossips about others to you will probably also gossip about you to others.

In general, it is best not to get involved in office gossip. Since nothing gets solved through idle talking, it is a waste of your time and energy and breeds low morale. Whether or not you have ADD, you can find more constructive ways to relax, gripe, or pass your time.

Occasionally, though, a conversation that starts off sounding like gossip can actually be an attempt to find out information that can be used constructively. How can you tell the difference?

When the same subject is talked about repeatedly and passed from one person to another without resolution, you can suspect gossiping. When personal matters are communicated that have nothing to do with job performance, you are also probably hearing gossip. Whenever you hear remarks prefaced by "Don't let so-and-so know I told you, but . . . ," you can be sure that gossip is in the air. Whining and complaining are typical of gossip. When all conversation stops when you walk into the room, you probably stepped into a gossip party. However, when a concerned coworker is overwhelmed and wants to talk out a situation, that's not gossip. When a person is upset and genuinely trying to figure out how to approach someone else, that's not gossip.

You'll know that you are the one doing the gossiping when you find yourself looking forward to the attention you anticipate from passing on a hot rumor. If you find you cannot hold other people's attention simply by sharing conversation but must think of something that either has shock value or is *about* someone else, you are probably gossiping. Finally, gossiping typically means you are telling what you have heard or think you know, not listening to another side of the story or trying to reach a solution.

You deserve to spend your time better than that, so use it for true communication with others, not gossip.

Working with a Team

Working with a team, a team in which each person contributes his or her own talents and skills, is often a great way to work—especially for people who have ADD. That way, the weaknesses that ADD can cause can be compensated for by the talents of others on the team. Furthermore, the special qualities that ADD brings can add tremendously to the team's creativity and problem-solving potential.

Teams have to be put together and worked out carefully. Ideally, team members who have ADD would have a healthy respect for their own strengths and weaknesses. No matter what, teamwork requires good communication and good relationships between team members.

Consider Dennis. Dennis, a hairstylist and teacher, always saw the big picture of whatever he was involved with. As a creative designer, his ideas were often far ahead of others'.

Yet, Dennis seemed to have very little ability to implement his ideas. For example, he had opportunities to put on large style shows periodically. Demonstrating techniques and teaching others was easy for him, but setting up the show felt like an overwhelming, if not impossible, task. He had no idea how to organize or even recognize the many details needed to get the show together, even though he had participated in many shows over the years. Because of his ADD, project management and keeping track of detailed plans were skills that had eluded him.

Dennis recognized the problem and hired others to plan the style shows for him. However, he had experienced more than one letdown when the people he had hired didn't follow through. His trust in others was shaken. Being unable to take over the job himself, he needed to depend on a trustworthy person, but who was trustworthy? How could he tell?

Dennis discovered that if he did not get regular feedback from the person he hired, he began to feel paranoid, suspecting that the person had changed his mind, didn't want to do the job anymore, or had run into an obstacle and wouldn't be able to complete the job. Dennis had to have specific, tangible communication from anyone he was working with so he would know how the project was coming. Otherwise, he became frightened and angry.

When Dennis became involved in any new relationship, he suffered fear and tended to put pressure on the other person until good lines of communication opened up. Then he could feel safe knowing that the work was being done—both his and the other person's. It was amazing how little he actually had to know in order to feel okay: just a word often sufficed.

Trouble would arise, however, when Dennis worked with someone who was insecure, like the time he teamed up with Larry. Larry assumed that Dennis didn't trust his work. Why else would Dennis be asking him so many questions about the work?

That was not at all the reason behind Dennis's need to know how the work was going. Obviously, Dennis and any partner or assistant had to talk out their individual needs and feelings of inadequacy before they could work comfortably together.

Betty and Gary teamed up to fulfill a mutual dream to have their own business. Both were interested in landscaping and were artistically inclined. Gary liked the physical aspect of putting in the landscaping, while Betty preferred organizing the projects and working with the finances. Both were good with people, but Betty was better at closing deals, while Gary liked building friendships with his customers.

It seemed like they were launching a successful venture until Betty discovered that Gary had failed to turn in paperwork at the end of the month—paperwork she needed in order to do the billing. Needless to say, she was not very happy. The business had bills to pay, little capital, and a poor cash flow. She began to see her dream dashed to bits.

Out of a sense of fear, Betty confronted Gary and accused him of being irresponsible. But Gary was bewildered. He thought he'd done exactly what she wanted; he certainly had intended to. He even remembered a conversation in which they had discussed billing. Betty had said, "Let me have your paperwork on the job regularly so I can do the billing. I've made arrangements with the buyers to divide their payments into three parts so we can have plenty of cash flow, since we're tight on money right now and need regular income."

In Betty's mind, the word "regularly" automatically meant "monthly." Because Gary has ADD and sees things in wholes rather than divided into arbitrary parts, he thought the word "regularly" meant after each job was completed. It never occurred to him to break a job up into parts that would be billed separately.

Betty, on the other hand, does not have ADD. She thinks of things in parts and pays attention to details. She had worked hard to develop a plan with which they would have a more even cash flow by billing customers monthly. It never occurred to her to specifically tell Gary that the individual jobs would be broken down into parts. Didn't everyone just do that automatically?

Fortunately, Gary did not get upset with Betty's accusations. He asked her to tell him specifically what she needed, when she needed it, and in what form. He reassured her that he was more than willing to comply, but he couldn't figure the process out unless she explained it, because he didn't think that way. When Betty realized that Gary thought about things differently than she and that he was very willing to do what she wanted, she relaxed and realized she needed to tell him in detail what she needed.

From then on they got along fine and did develop a successful, smoothly running business, built on mutual respect for each other's differences, cooperation, and good communication.

The Benefits of Working with an ADD Team Member

People with ADD do very well teaming up with non-ADD coworkers. For example, there's the charismatic person with Outwardly Expressive ADD who enchants and sells customers on the technical innovations of a quiet, introverted inventor. Without such a highly charged, motivated member of the team, the greatest technical achievement could lie dormant, unused, and unrewarded.

People with Inwardly Expressive ADD tend to be creative dreamers and may also be very good listeners and great friends, due to their sensitivity. In combination with a partner who has a high public profile, such a person may be a hidden but active part of creative successes. This type of partnership may be represented publicly by the partner with the higher profile, but in reality there are people working behind the scenes to bring the creations to fruition.

We've all heard people say, "I couldn't have done it without my wife [or husband]." You can take this to heart regardless of how smart, skilled, or talented the speaker may be. No one can do everything.

One young man I know, though a talented photographer, is even more skilled as a friend and team member. Mike taught me how to network and how to be a team member, not just as the leader but as a full-fledged teammate.

As I watched what he did that drew people to him, I saw that, first of all, he listened. He always seemed to have time for someone who needed him, and he made the person feel as if she and what she had to say was the most important thing in the world. Mike not only listens; he affirms what the other person desires to do. Then he makes suggestions to help that person reach her goal. He makes trades of services and products, bringing people together.

Before I knew it, using Mike's teachings, I found myself surrounded by people who were eager and willing to help me with my dreams, and I found we had much to give one another. Mike's role on the team was to keep us connected. He kept the team vibrant by continuing the process of bringing new people in when their skills were needed or their interests coincided with those of the rest of us.

Negotiating with a Team

Any interpersonal relationship requires give-and-take, compromise, and, usually, negotiation. That's because the purpose of a team is to combine skills and talents. If the team did everything the way one member wanted, there wouldn't be much purpose for the team members to have gotten together in the first place.

Having ADD can sometimes complicate those compromises and negotiations. For example, if you have Highly Structured ADD, negotiation can be quite difficult because you tend to see things in black-and-white, right-or-wrong terms.

Terry's job as chief financial officer required that he bring comparative construction costs to meetings. Diagnosed with primarily the Highly Structured form of ADD, Terry had a perspective where only one thing mattered: the bottom line. No matter what anyone else had to say, if the finances didn't mesh, Terry argued against it.

When his work team was faced with the task of deciding where and how to construct a new shopping center, he discovered how stressful being one of six members on a team could be for him. Imagine his dismay when the vice-president in charge of expansion, a person with Outwardly Expressive ADD, flamboyantly announced that this shopping center was to be a model for future development over the next ten years—and cost was no object. The architect envisioned magnificent design plans that would place the center not only ahead of the local competition but make it state of the art.

Terry immediately positioned himself in an adversarial role with the other team members. He would not hear them out and help them find ways to achieve at least some of what they wanted while still holding costs under control. Meeting after meeting ended in someone walking out with no progress made. Eventually, the project was scrapped, and the company retreated to maintaining its existing enterprises, falling behind in the marketplace. The vice president and the project architect left the company to go into partnership together. Terry was offered early retirement, because, many say, he just could not work well on a team.

The flip side is that power struggles can bring out the best in everyone when they work to arrive at a consensus. Consensus is quite different from compromise, in which no one really gets exactly what he wants. With consensus, everyone agrees to find ways that please everyone else without anyone losing. There are no power struggles, and no winners or losers emerge.

Daryl, a valuable employee, worked for a nonprofit organization as its public information officer. For personal reasons, he wanted to move to a country setting where the business did not have an office. He went to his boss to see whether something could be worked out. Each of them listened to the other outline his needs and desires. Neither interrupted. When they finished, Daryl's boss said, "Okay. I want to keep you as an employee. You want to move but would also like to continue to do the work you are doing for us. Let's figure out how to make that happen."

Together they noticed that almost all of Daryl's work was already done via computer, fax, and telephone. He traveled with his job, but the new location had access to an airport, and he found out it would not cost the company any more to fly out of that airport than the current one. Also, little need existed for Daryl and his boss to meet face to face.

Though Daryl's boss did not know that Daryl had ADD, he did know that Daryl was a talented writer, communicator, and negotiator. He knew that Daryl's sensitivity to others made him an excellent representative for the organization. Yet, he realized that Daryl had been uncomfortable in the office for some time, because Daryl had remarked how distracted he was during the workday by all the activity. In fact, Daryl often took his work home or came in early when he had key assignments due that took thoughtful preparation.

Together they concluded that Daryl could live in the location he desired, work out of his home, and still do the job they both would like him to do. The boss realized that Daryl's living in the new area could actually solve some problems, such as office noise, that had plagued him from the very beginning. In this situation, retention of a valuable employee resulted from their negotiations.

"He Looks Great, but . . ."

People with ADD, especially people with Outwardly Expressive ADD, are often seen by those who do not have to work with them as wonderful. They are known for their charisma and high profile, which can make others look forward to working with them. For short periods of time this illusion continues, but given time for paperwork to pile up, late assignments to accumulate, moodiness or tempers to erupt, or sensitive feelings to get stepped on, the luster wears off. When the person working closely with the ADD individual then tries to improve the work situation, she may be ignored, rejected, or told she's making too much of nothing.

Malcolm's charisma as a minister drew new people to his small church every week. Only recently hired, he was enjoying his popularity. He seemed to be the answer to everyone's prayers. After a few months, though, one person did not share in that general consensus: Malcolm's secretary. She knew how he threw the newsletter and Sunday program together at the last minute. She paid the price daily when people called up needing paperwork that only the minister could deliver. Budgets, plans, and copy for the board of directors' meetings were nowhere to be found. More often than she liked, she had to cover for his tardiness or make excuses when he forgot to keep an appointment. She knew what really existed behind the closed doors of his office: stacks and stacks of papers, so much that he had ceased meeting with people there and took them into a small prayer room that was kept paper-free.

When the secretary tried to get help from the president of the board of directors, she was told that she was making too much of the situation, that he was the best minister the church had ever had, and that no one was perfect. She talked to the minister himself and shared her concern. He laughed and said he never had been very good with details, but that he'd try harder. Besides, that was why he needed her so much.

But nothing changed. Frustrated, she stopped trying to talk about the problem. Ten months later, an outside audit by the national church discovered that the business affairs were in total chaos and that the church was ready to fold financially. Though a popular preacher, this minister with ADD could not run a church. Only the one who worked close to him had known it.

Working with Support Staff

Many people with ADD get along particularly well with support staff, such as maintenance workers, minimum-wage employees, and temporary help. If you have Outwardly Expressive ADD, you probably have a gift of gab and find yourself talking with the president of the company and the janitor with equal ease. Outgoing and nonjudgmental, you tend to see the value in everyone's contribution to the job.

If your ADD is primarily Inwardly Directed, you will probably gravitate to people with similar skills and talents who can talk about or enjoy the skills you have to offer. For example, as a potter, Joyce could spend all day talking with the supplier of her clay, and she loved to talk with the deliveryman who set up her new kiln and loves his job of pleasing craftsmen by doing a top-notch job of installation.

Kennedy's father was an auto mechanic, his brother is one, and now Kennedy is learning to be one. Though quiet in many settings, when he gets around shops, auto parts people, auto wholesalers, and vintage car buffs, he opens up, talking about pistons, wind resistance, and tire treads. He appreciates anyone who has anything to do with cars—whether it's the supervisor of the parts department or the after-hours crew that cleans the offices—and lets them know it. Predictably, Kennedy is very well liked.

In his brother's shop the janitor waits until Kennedy finishes for the day so they can talk together about cars and about Kennedy's dream of hiring onto a race-car team. Even though the janitor is a slow learner, Kennedy values the time they spend together not just because he has an audience, but because his empathy for others draws him to a man who is doing all he can do with the limited resources he has—and also loves to talk about cars. Kennedy really sees the best in everyone.

Sometimes, though, people who have ADD can be offensive to support staff without meaning to be. They get caught up in a whirlwind of activity, overlooking anyone who isn't immediately visible to them on the job. Unaware of details, some people with ADD have no idea what it takes to get a complicated show on the road. Consequently, paying no attention to the many intricate aspects of completing a project, they may fail to say, "Thank you," to the support staff who held everything together so that the ADD person could do his thing.

If You're Self-Employed

A disproportionately large number of people who have ADD choose to go into business for themselves, relative to people who do not have

ADD. This is partly because of the entrepreneurial spirit inherent in the way in which you are wired and partly because of the excitement of taking a risk doing something new. People with ADD are very likely to be creative and have a strong desire to do things in their own way. Consequently, self-employment often suits the talents and gifts of people with ADD. (See Chapter 9.)

Even if you are in business for yourself, though, you still have to deal with other people. Just as if you were someone else's employee, maybe even more so, your interpersonal skills may make or break your success. You need to get along with customers, suppliers, staff, your banker, your accountant, the IRS, a landlord, and the kid who wants to hang around your shop.

When you work for someone else, the only person you *must* get along with is your boss. It's true that he or she may be influenced by how well you get along with others, but unless you are terribly offensive, you may simply be considered eccentric or hard to get along with.

With your own business, however, your sphere of influence is much greater. You are in competition with others who have similar businesses, and your customers can go elsewhere. You are dependent on many people. If you don't treat suppliers right, they can quit cooperating with you, deny you favors when you most need them, or refuse to deal with you altogether. The bank may give you a hard time or refuse to give you what you need. Neighborhood vandals may even pick you out because you are a "mean person."

Obviously, the way around these problems is to "make friends and influence people." Remember first and foremost that these relationships are voluntary and, consequently, different from those you may have had as an employee. Then keep in mind that you must not only cultivate good working relationships with the many people you encounter, but you must keep them.

Right now, make a list of the people you are dependent upon in order to do your business. You may be surprised at how long it is. After each name put a number that stands for your evaluation of how well you and the person communicate. Make "1" stand for "poorly" and "5" stand for "great." Consider each person on the list and ask whether you have any unfinished business with that person, hurt feelings, anger, a misunderstanding, or confusion. How are you doing?

Most importantly, commit to doing something about what you find. You may wish to go to the persons and ask for clarification. Whatever you do, don't let confusion remain. Communicate your feelings, not with a long list of complaints, unless things are really bad, but simply and concisely. Discuss what happened. Ask each person if his or her intent was to make you angry or hurt. Then tell that person what you need in order to feel all right about the situation. Make your request short.

When Tim, a cafe owner, received the last drop-off of produce three days in a row, he became upset. Not only was it not very fresh, but because the shipment came so late, he had had to buy some other produce at retail prices to get started for the day. On top of that, when his order came, it did not contain all the produce he'd ordered. He called the supplier, told him what had happened, and asked why this was happening. The supplier apologized, saying that he was short one truck and driver and had to redistribute the amount sent out on each route.

Tim said he either wanted to be served earlier in the delivery process or be assured that he would get plenty of fresh fruit and vegetables in a timely manner. When the supplier jumped in and agreed to Tim's request, Tim did not feel the need to threaten the man by saying, "Either meet my request, or I'll change suppliers." By working with the man when he was in a difficult situation, Tim not only received what he wanted but won the man's respect and had a favor in the bank to call upon when he needed one.

Ironically, it wasn't very long until Tim needed to call on that favor. He ran into a temporary cash flow problem because of remodeling and needed a few days' extension on the payment of some of his bills. The first person he thought about asking was the produce supplier. Sure enough the man said, "No problem. You worked with me; I'll work with you."

In contrast, think about how harmful it is to relationships if you have a temper that causes you to blow up before you have time to think things over. Imagine the repercussions of blaming others without getting both sides of the story. When you work on any of these ADD-related traits that can cause big interpersonal problems, you'll be a lot better off in business for yourself: temper, oversensitivity, over-reactivity to stress, impulsivity (both verbal and physical), listening and other communication deficits, organizational difficulties, impatience, and inattention to other's needs and feelings.

Self-Protection and Setting Limits

When you own your own business, you must be self-protective. No one else will step in to do the job for you. William made a mistake, one that people with ADD often make: he put too much trust in a person who promised to market his wares but actually did little. Innocently, William kept making payments to the person until finally he realized that no business was forthcoming.

William had had a feeling earlier that this relationship was not working, but he believed the marketer when he said things would change as soon as some of the problems were out of the way. Instead, though, problems just kept surfacing. William ended up losing quite a bit of money because he neither set limits ahead of time nor trusted his intuition.

Naively, many people with ADD are so used to overworking and feeling inadequate that they give much more than half to relationships that should be fifty-fifty. In the end, someone is able to take advantage of them because they did not set limits and protect themselves. Learning to be watchful and valuing what you have to offer is your best protection in such situations.

Romance on the Job

In any work situation involving adults, an office romance can develop. If you've ever been involved in that type of romance or watched a coworker become involved in one, you probably know how tricky it can be—whether or not you have ADD.

If you do have ADD, however, the odds are even higher for you than your non-ADD coworker that you may get involved romantically at work, primarily because of your empathy and sensitivity to others. If you have Outwardly Expressive ADD, you tend to act your feelings out, expressing yourself so that everyone around you knows what your heart is saying. Loving to talk, caring about others, and enjoying the charisma that you have makes you attractive to others, both platonically and sexually.

Because you are a kinesthetic person, learning by doing, you tend to try things out before spending much time thinking about them. All forms of ADD have this characteristic. Of course, that means you are more likely to get involved with someone than the average person. The two of you discover how you feel, how you work together, and what you like about each other by spending time together. Spending that time together creates an environment in which romance can easily blossom.

Being verbally impulsive also contributes to romantic involvement. There you go—without thinking—saying and doing what your heart feels rather than what your logical mind tells you is the sensible thing to do. Before you know it, you're involved.

For example, consider Hector and Marguerite, both of whom have ADD. They were assigned to the same station after boot camp. In the clerical pool, since they were both newcomers, they quickly turned to one another for support. Both felt overwhelmed by the new environment in which they found themselves, just like many people with ADD, who often take longer to adjust to new situations than their non-ADD counterparts.

Eager to feel better, they began talking about what was happening and how they felt about it. They each discovered that the other was sensitive, which was most appealing. They felt as if they had known one another for a long time, and they quickly became romantically and sexually involved. For a while, they couldn't seem to get enough of each other.

Then two things happened. First, Marguerite was promoted faster than Hector because she was better able to follow through with her work. Also, Hector had a more explosive temper, which that did not endear him to his superiors. Second, Marguerite was able to become comfortable on the job faster than Hector, and she wanted to do things other than talk about work.

Marguerite began to get tired of Hector's constant complaining, and she discovered that he had developed few interests growing up. Though neither had worked up to their potential in school, Marguerite had spent more time with outside interests and developed her love for sports and volunteering. She wanted to continue with these interests, but Hector seemed to only be able to complain about work.

Hector's complaining finally bothered Marguerite so much that she told him she didn't love him anymore and wanted to stop seeing him exclusively. She planned to do things with her time off that involved other people. Hector's temper flared. Already feeling inadequate and angry, he hounded Marguerite. Because they worked together, she was never free of his irritating snipes, rude remarks, and threats. Finally, she had to request a transfer in order to get away from Hector.

A romantic breakup with someone at work almost always creates problems. Hurt or angry feelings, such as those between Marguerite and Hector, are hard to ignore when you are thrown together daily. Even if you try to ignore your feelings, your coworkers can feel the tension they create. It's not always easy or desirable to make a job change just so you can get away from the other person.

Yet, being thrown together on a team or simply working closely together with someone else creates warm feelings. It's natural to want to become involved with someone, especially if you are excited about your work or have overcome work-related problems. If you don't have a good rein on your emotions, it's easy to begin to express the affection you feel when you are romantically attracted to your coworker.

How Susceptible Are You to Romance on the Job?

Would you like to know whether you are a prime candidate to become romantically involved at work? Ask yourself these questions: Do you fall in love "at the drop of a hat"? Do you give your whole heart to someone who treats you nicely? Are you impulsive when your sexual feelings are stirred? Do you tend to use sex to feel better about yourself or to relieve tension? Do you get sexual feelings confused with being creative, excited, or expressive, thinking it is sexual energy you're feeling rather than creative excitement?

If you answer positively to any of these questions, be careful. You may be mixing up sexual feelings with the pleasure that comes from working closely with someone else. You may also want to ask yourself whether you have ever had close work friends with whom you *haven't* been romantically involved. If you've not had this kind of experience, it would be worth your while to cultivate such a friend.

You are also at high risk to have an affair on the job if your current marriage or committed relationship is in trouble. The most natural thing in the world is to look around for a substitute, but I promise you, this is not the time to allow one to develop. Watch out for such a relationship to *just happen*. I can't tell you how many times I've heard those words. Rarely do these relationships work out. But if, in fact, you have found the perfect mate at such a time, that relationship will endure through a waiting period.

Having affairs simply doesn't work, ever. I'm not talking from a moral standpoint but a psychological one. By having an affair with someone at work, you continually dilute the relationship because you are playing two roles with the person. Consequently, you don't have to fully face either the personal or the work relationship. Not only do affairs compromise your performance on the job—even though at first you may be excited, energized, and more productive than normal—but they pull people down because of needing to keep the secret.

If you are in a poor relationship with someone, end it before starting another. Know that you can never know what a new one will really be like if you are still in an old one. An affair usually allows a person not to have to deal with either relationship fully. If a divorce happens, the affair often also falls apart because of the full availability of the now-divorced partner.

Even if your logical side agrees with this advice, we all know that avoiding romance at work is not always easy. How can you keep from becoming involved? First, become clear with yourself that your work and personal lives are separate. Know why you are at work. When you find yourself working with someone, realize that the possibility always exists that you might become attracted romantically. Pay attention to both your feelings and your behavior. If you begin to feel eager to spend time with the person, recognize your feelings. If you do favors for the person, try to find ways to be around the person, or note that you want to get close or even touch the other person, become aware that you may be developing special feelings for him or her.

Also pay attention when you notice similar behavior coming from someone else. Don't just brush it aside or tell yourself, "Oh, no, he couldn't possibly be interested in me." Pay attention to it.

Such feelings and desires are absolutely normal and healthy, but having them doesn't mean that you need to let them take over. Just notice them in yourself or the other person and acknowledge them.

Often, such attraction can simply be handled with humor. You may want to kid around a little bit saying something like, "You're just the kind of guy I'd like to get to know in my next life," or "Hey, gorgeous, wanna boogie?" And off you go on a joint sales call, laughing. You both know you're just kidding around. Yes, you feel affection for one another, but you're communicating that neither of you intends to go any further with the relationship.

Sometimes, though, you have to have a more serious talk, one that sets the record straight and gives both of you guidelines to follow. You might want to say, "I've really been enjoying working with you. I've also noticed that I have some feelings that are not just work related, but I don't want to mix work and pleasure, so I need to talk with you a little about this." Then wait to get a reaction, which could be anything from stark surprise to acknowledgment that the other person has the same feelings.

Remember that if the other person does not feel the same way you do, there is nothing to be ashamed of. Your feelings are wonderful, and they are yours. Do not let them get them hurt because of lack of reciprocity. Simply say, "Thanks for listening. I'm an emotional person who has strong feelings about what I like, and I appreciate your being in my life. Now I can concentrate better on the job we're doing."

If it turns out that the other person shares your feelings, you both need to determine what you want to do with them. A lot of the decision will depend on whether you both are free to enter into a new personal relationship. If one or both of you is not personally free, I strongly recommend that you do not get involved. If you both are free and you want to explore the possibility, talk about the implications on the job if things don't work out. Commit to keep your romancing outside of the workplace. And agree to be honest with one another.

I would recommend that you assess yourself and the other person in terms of stability. If someone is very emotionally erratic and seems to experience intense highs or lows, be aware that disappointment will be experienced keenly. Go slowly and carefully. If you choose to become emotionally involved, you should realize now that if things don't work out, you may have to change your job or job setting. Ask yourself whether you are willing to do that. Then proceed with care.

Set boundaries of what you will and will not do about your feelings in the work setting. Be clear and stick to your decisions. Remember, rushing into a relationship, or pressuring someone else to move quickly in a relationship, is a sure sign that fear or insecurity lies underneath. Take it easy, use good common sense to temper your feelings, and enjoy one another in a leisurely manner. You are likely to save both the relationship and the job with this approach.

6

The Boss and Other Authority Issues

Good Boss versus Bad Boss

Heard any great "bad boss" stories lately? Sure you have. Everyone has a story about a boss whose demands are outrageous, or a boss who didn't give a raise in five years, and so on. Bad boss stories are everywhere. Anyone who's been in the workplace for any amount of time has a bad boss story, so we know this is not just an issue for people with ADD. No one likes being bossed around. No one likes feeling that his or her work isn't appreciated. If you plan to stay employed for any amount of time, however, you will have to deal with the fact that someone will have authority over your work and over your job. Fortunately, not all bosses are bad.

What Makes a Good Boss?

Dorothy's job as a clerical worker in a large corporation changed when she was assigned to a new boss. Her work load increased drastically, but she didn't say anything for a while, thinking she just had to get used to the new situation. However, after several months Dorothy realized things weren't getting any better, so she explained to her boss that the amount of work he was giving her simply couldn't be done by one person.

Her boss responded with a surprised yet accepting expression and told Dorothy how glad he was that she had come to him. He had no idea that the problem existed. He asked Dorothy to do two things. First, he wanted a list of the duties she could reasonably accomplish. He suggested that she choose ones she preferred to do. Then he wanted a list of the duties that she would like to see a second person take over. He also asked her to consider whether it would take a full-time or part-time second person to do those jobs. He told Dorothy he was going to try get another employee to help out, but if he couldn't, they'd work something else out. He then set a time for them to meet again in two days.

When they met the second time, he not only acknowledged the excellent job she'd been doing but again apologized for overloading her. Even better, much to Dorothy's relief, he immediately agreed to implement the selections she'd made. He thanked her for letting him know of the problem and encouraged her to feel free to come to him at any time in the future if she had anything on her mind. He also asked her to keep an eye on the work flow and let him know how it was going, and he suggested they touch base in a month.

Even if another employee could not have been added, Dorothy's boss was prepared to continue to problem-solve the overload so that Dorothy didn't have to pay the price. He would have told her that it was his job to figure this out with her and that he appreciated her patience. Dorothy has a good boss.

What Makes a Bad Boss?

Two kinds of bad bosses make life miserable for employees. The first kind is well-meaning but inept. Carrie had that kind of boss. Disorganized and inattentive, with his hand in many pies, her boss dropped work on her desk day and night. If she said anything, he responded with, "Oh, I know you can get to it. You're great."

But Carrie couldn't get to it. As the stress built, she asked her boss for a time when they could meet. He said he'd get back to her on it, but he didn't. When she reminded him, her boss simply said, "I've been too busy, but let's meet tomorrow." When tomorrow came, however, her boss was out of town on a business trip. He'd failed to check his calendar when making the appointment. On returning, he apologized, but three months later they still hadn't met. Things were still haphazard, and Carrie continued to be overworked. Though a nice guy, her boss was thoughtless, was a poor organizer, and didn't follow through on his promises.

The other type of bad boss is one who is just plain mean and, frankly, has no business bossing anyone. Torrance had that kind of boss.

Arrogant and foul-mouthed, his boss continually put Torrance down. "If you can't cut the mustard, leave. There are ten more people standing in line for your job. I don't have time to mess around with someone who is always complaining."

Torrance's boss even went behind his back, talking about how inadequate he was and how stressful it was to have to work with someone who couldn't get the job done. Needless to say, Torrance's self-esteem took a beating, and there was no reasoning with his boss.

Torrance's boss was not workable. He was so caught up in his own needs, and he was so down on others who had lower work status than him, that he couldn't treat them with respect. Without respect for your value and skills, no employee can function effectively or feel good about himself.

Bosses automatically have power over employees. They also have more responsibility. Because the buck stops at the boss's feet, a good boss takes and expresses as much power as he or she has responsibility, not more nor less.

Bad bosses use power to meet their own needs rather than to meet their responsibilities on the job. Good bosses consider themselves responsible for certain things and also manage to respect the job done by those who work under them. Together they form a team. A bad boss doesn't know how or want to work on a team.

The Best Bosses: The ADD Perspective

From your perspective as someone with ADD, this authority stuff on a personal and emotional level either makes you or breaks you. Being oversensitive to authority and responding poorly to it can turn your work into a tiresome chore or, at worst, into a nightmare. You've no doubt experienced both.

On a tangible level, your perspective will get you either hired or fired. Ultimately, getting along with your boss, regardless of whether that person is right or what is done is fair, dictates your success on the job. So, you'd better get real good at getting along with that person, or figure out the time has come to look elsewhere for employment.

The best boss, with characteristics that generally work well with employees who are ADD, can be described as follows:

▪ Someone who asks people to do specific tasks, instead of ordering them

- Someone who has some structure and order in his or her own life
- Someone who presents material in an orderly way
- Someone who is regular and predictable, even in his or her response to a crisis situation
- Someone who can clearly express his or her expectations
- Someone who respects others, valuing differences
- Someone who is nonjudgmental
- Someone who looks at his or her employees' skills, then tries to fit the job to the person, or encourages the person to consider a more appropriate job within the company

The Best Boss for Someone with Outwardly Expressive ADD

If you have the form of ADD that is Outwardly Expressive, you are likely to be very outgoing, expressive, and sure of what you want. You will benefit from a boss who sets limits in a supportive, not suffocating, way. Because you have trouble setting limits on yourself, you can often benefit from some structure that ensures you'll finish. That way you can reach your dreams and goals. These limits, though, need to be along the lines that feel right to you.

Anthony loved his job as a stand-up comic. He worked for an entertainment company that got him bookings. His boss recognized and understood the value of Anthony's talents and creativity. He also realized that Anthony had a tendency to agree to any request made of him, which meant that Anthony was often running in twenty directions at once. Starting many ventures, Anthony rarely made much money because he didn't follow through on the most promising leads.

So his boss set some limits on Anthony, saying, "You're so talented, Anthony, that I hate to see you missing out on the success you can make in this business. From here on out, I want us to meet weekly to go over all the leads you've received. We'll decide which ones to follow up on and which ones to let go. Then you can finish the ones we've selected, and you can begin to make some more money for yourself. You'll be able to work smarter. Will you do it?"

It was very important that the boss ask Anthony if he would be willing to work within the limits. If he'd automatically imposed them,

Anthony would have resisted. Anthony quickly recognized how much his boss was trying to help him, being on his team to do something for him that he couldn't do for himself. Everyone wins.

Victoria, a sharp salesperson, finally found the boss who could give her what she needed. Mr. Corbett, as he liked to be called, seemed a bit aloof to Victoria at first, but she quickly came to realize that she benefited from his calm, methodical way of dealing with her. He not only assigned someone to help her with her appointments and paperwork, but he spoke with her reassuringly first thing every day. Only after a few months did it dawn on her that he was actually calming her down every morning so that she could focus better on what she was going to do for the day. He would nonchalantly go over the prospects she had set up. Then he'd say something like, "I'm really glad that you're going to be finalizing the Schultz deal and checking back on First Bank." Even if Victoria had forgotten something that he had brought up, she didn't have to lose face by being "caught." Instead, she could receive his reminders in a supportive environment that didn't drain her emotionally.

After working for Mr. Corbett for a year, Victoria discovered that she had adopted many of his mannerisms. She often heard him talking in her mind, reminding her to do something. He had truly shaped her behavior, making her a more effective salesperson. He was perfect for her.

The best boss for Frank in chapter two would be one who could help Frank feel appreciated while setting a firm limit on his temper. All the boss really would need to do would be to start any conversation with, "You're important to me. I need your help." He'd have Frank in the palm of his hand.

If Frank walked off in a fit of temper, a good boss for him would let him go. Then, when Frank returned, he could say, "I'm glad you're back. Look, let's talk about what happened. I want to know your side of the story." Later, after the whole incident was done and forgotten, his boss could call Frank aside in private and say, "Frank, I need you around here. I trust you and your work, but I don't like you blowing up. Would you be willing to work on it? If you are, I'll help you. Come to me when you feel mad. I'll stop what I'm doing, if I can, and you can learn to talk about what's bothering you rather than just blowing up. Deal?"

Bosses of people with Outwardly Expressive ADD need to clear the way for this type of person to "do their thing." By setting an effective framework in place, best use of the person's talents leads to improved productivity and satisfaction on the job. A calm, firm hand and asking rather than telling are essential. Though people with this form of ADD may appear in control and confident, don't ever forget how very sensitive they are.

Best Boss for Someone with Inwardly Expressive ADD

As someone whose ADD is quietly expressed, you probably tend to prefer bosses who give you your assignment, then leave you alone. You are quite possibly artistically or mechanically talented, and expression comes through the demonstration of your skills. A boss who gives you work that fits those talents, gives you, him, and the job a favor.

Moriah does design work for a pottery company that specializes in individualized orders. She hates her new boss, who expects her to cover the front counter when the salesperson is out. She'll probably quit, even though she used to love her job. Her old boss understood that she needed to be left alone to do her creative work and made sure that someone else was always available to handle customers. Moriah needs that protection to feel good about her job.

People with Type II ADD are generally not complainers, so their bosses would do well to touch base regularly, asking how things are going. They then need to wait for an answer. By giving a little encouragement, the boss can probably gain useful information to pinpoint some problem areas in the workplace. Quietness should not be misunderstood to mean this type of person doesn't see what's going on. A good boss knows that. Furthermore, he listens carefully to any complaints because an Inwardly Directed person probably doesn't say anything until the work problem has gotten quite big.

Another trait of Inwardly Directed people is the tendency to get stuck in situations. When Claudio's boss noticed that he had been working for two days on an electrical problem with a customer's car he said, "Let's just pack it away for now. I need you to work on the sedan that just came in. You can go back later and try again." Claudio needed his boss to help him stop for now. He'd always had trouble with his "record" getting stuck. Probably later, with a fresh eye, he'd see something in the first car that he'd overlooked.

Inwardly Directed people need support, guidelines, and protection in order to do what they do well. They also need encouragement to verbalize what's wrong so they don't stuff their feelings inside. Their hypersensitivity can be masked behind the lack of expressiveness and result in depression. A skillful boss recognizes this and makes it easy for the Type

II person to get things off his or her chest.

The Best Boss for Someone with Highly Structured ADD

A good boss for the person with Type III ADD is precise, clear, and straightforward. Preferably, they are in a work setting that changes little, where a structure that doesn't vary is in place. If the job does not naturally have a tight structure, it is the boss's responsibility to put one in place.

When Chester took over the job as chief financial officer for a new computer company, he discovered that the company had grown quickly because of the creative genius of a young owner, but every aspect of the business was in disarray. Chester quickly became frustrated.

However, a new chief executive officer was brought in who saved the day for Chester and the company. The CEO made the structuring of Chester's job his top priority. He laid out guidelines for Chester's areas of responsibility and set limits on other administrative staff, so Chester knew exactly what was expected of him and what he could count on from others.

Because people with Highly Structured ADD tend to be uncompromising, judging things to be right or wrong, they often do not make very good team members. Nancy's boss did not expect her to be a part of a work team at the beginning of a project, so she and the team were spared from going through the brainstorming, negotiation stage together. Instead, she was called in for her expertise when the team had specific questions for her or needed the solution to a particular problem that called for her skills. Nancy liked it that way, and her boss made sure it happened. The rest of the time, Nancy simply pursued her projects on her own.

Change is very hard for Highly Structured Ned. When he decided to leave the military, he tried to find a pilot job that would suit his desire to do things precisely and within familiar guidelines. He decided to take a job temporarily with a small airline that ferried freight until he could get on with a major carrier. Ned's boss understood his needs but could not meet them because of the irregular demands for service. Some weeks Ned flew back-to-back flights. Other times he sat around waiting for the next flight. He couldn't plan anything with regularity, and it made him anxious. When his boss needed him to quickly change his schedule because of an unplanned cutback, Ned blew up. His boss, realizing that the job didn't fit Ned, recommended that he do something else until he could get the regular job he wanted.

Ned took a temporary job selling precision machinery parts to specialty shops. His expertise was appreciated, and his hours were regular, with no unexpected changes. Ned felt much better and was able to manage, even though his pay was much lower than previously, until eventually being hired by an airline. The last I heard, he was doing fine and liked working within the familiar limits provided by a regular flight schedule over which he had some control.

Power Struggles: The Power of the Job Title versus Emotional Power

Power Comes with the Title of Boss

Let's be realistic: every boss has some tangible power, or he or she wouldn't be "the boss." Unless you work for yourself, you will have a boss. Even the CEO has a board of directors looking over his shoulder. And inherent in the title of *boss* is power and authority.

The kind of power I'm talking about affects your being hired, fired, promoted, and assigned to tasks. Whether your boss is right or wrong, fair or tyrannical, does not matter. As long as that person is your boss, you are helpless to do much that the person disagrees with. In the real world, the boss usually wins out because of his power.

Even with government help such as through the Equal Employment Opportunities Commission (EEOC) and the Americans with Disabilities Act (ADA), your life can be made pretty miserable trying to overcome the influence wielded by your boss. Although in the long run you may have a case, you'd better like adversarial conditions if you are going to go up against the power of a boss.

Ultimately, your boss influences not just your current job but your career. The way in which you work out your differences may haunt you. You can't just blow up at the boss as you might a coworker. Nor can you simply do your own thing. Understand exactly what kind of power your boss's job entitles him or her to, and you will have much better control over your career or job.

Define and Talk about Emotional Power

Emotional power is different from the power inherent in the title *boss*. Emotional power is within you and determines your ability to get your own needs met within the limits of the outside power around you. Earlier in this book I've talked a lot about asking for help. If you need help and do not ask for it, you are failing to act powerfully to get what you need.

Emotional power also involves setting limits on what you will and won't do. It protects you. If you do something a coworker tells you to that you don't want to do, you give your power away to that person. To act powerfully, you need to say no when you don't want to do something.

A boss has tangible power over you, and you may not be able to say no to her without jeopardizing your position. You can say, "I'll do it if I must, but I'd rather not," or "Is there someone else who could do the job?" If you end up accepting the assignment because no one else can do it, you have still acted powerfully by exploring the limits around your boss's request.

A boss's emotional power needs to be as great as his job power, or he's likely to abuse the power attached to his job. Policemen, for example, have large amounts of power and authority because of the nature of their job. Often, however, a cop "goes wrong" because the power given to him creates temptations.

Eunice took great pride in her police uniform. Graduating at the top of her class, she'd wanted to work for the force since she was small child. The thought of wearing a badge made her feel safe after being raised in a chaotic household, where her father's drinking terrified her and her sisters. The oldest girl, she became a perfectly behaved child and model student, but inside she felt very angry about her home life.

Her supervisor began to notice that Eunice not only took pride in her uniform but seemed to talk a lot about how much authority she had. "Nobody better mess with me tonight. I'll show them who's boss." Having been on the force for a long time, her supervisor noticed the signs of an officer whose emotional power was weaker than the power inherent in her job. He referred her for psychological counseling, before real trouble could erupt. Eventually, Eunice became a successful policewoman, after she overcame the fear and pain she'd suffered as a child and was truly able to grow into an emotionally powerful woman.

All managers must have as much or more emotional power than their employees, or trouble is sure to follow. Quintan, a sales manager for a major hotel chain, had twelve people working for him—and a wishy-washy way of doing business. He'd tell a salesman to do something, but when it went undone, he wouldn't do anything about it. Also, he often didn't do what he said he would do.

Most of his employees were more emotionally powerful than he. No one respected Quintan. His staff called him irresponsible and laughed behind his back. They pretty much did what they wanted to do and looked for ways to aggravate him. Morale was low, and business suffered. When confronted by his supervisors, Quintan blamed the lack of sales on his salesmen, saying they wouldn't do anything he told them to do.

Signs of low emotional power include irresponsibility, bullying, setting one person against another, using threats, picking on people, not being direct, acting helpless, lying, and failing to set or enforce limits. When you learn to recognize these in people you work for and with, you'll begin to have an idea about what to do. Often the person who appears to be the biggest bully or blowhard is actually the most afraid, whether that person is your boss or a coworker.

It's hard to respect a boss who does not handle power well, but you don't have to sink to his or her level of powerlessness yourself. By focusing your attention on the tasks at hand, being assertive but not pushy, and asking for clarification when the other person misuses power, you can survive until you either get a different boss or decide to make a change.

Clara eventually decided to change jobs when her boss continually failed to support her. As a news reporter for a major television station, she frequently found herself privy to stories that were controversial but good for ratings. She followed procedure by going to her boss with an outline of a situation and her plan for covering the story. It was up to him to give his approval for her to go ahead.

However, too often after Clara had gained his approval and done a top-notch job, her boss would fail to support her when controversy surfaced. Finally, when she and the station were sued because of a true but touchy subject, she knew it was time to find a new boss because her boss said, "I can't imagine why she pursued this so adamantly." Fortunately for her, she had witnesses who presented evidence of the truth of her story, and eventually the suit was dropped. She was tired of the problem of working for an emotionally powerless boss, though, and took power into her own hands: She changed jobs.

Authority Issues Related to the ADD Employee

A lifetime of doing things differently and often being criticized because of it have left many ADD people painfully sensitive to being criticized and judged. You are already extremely sensitive because of your ADD, with the result that you are vulnerable to the evaluations and critiques that are a part of every job.

Impulsivity, also a natural aspect of being ADD, can mar your performance and undermine relations with superiors and coworkers. Add a hot temper to the mix, and you are set up to do something that is not self-promoting. Getting your behavior under control, especially managing your emotions around authority, makes the time you spend on the job much more pleasant and productive.

Hypersensitivity

When you see, smell, taste, and hear things more acutely than the average person, your hypersensitivity is showing. Your sense of touch is also likely to be highly developed. You are also likely blessed with an inner sense that allows you to experience with your own feelings what is going on inside other people. You therefore pick up others' disapproval, fear, and anger easily, though you may not know where the feelings are coming from. You often intuitively know what is going to happen before it happens because you *sense* something is "on the wind."

Being hypersensitive means you just have lots of sensitivity, which you can use as an asset as well as a liability. Your hypersensitivity is neither good nor bad: it just is. However, before you learn to manage your sensitive feelings, they can cause you considerable pain. Your boss can make you feel worse by not recognizing that you are as sensitive as you are. On the other hand, your boss can make your life a whole lot easier by helping you work with your sensitivity.

Jamie and LaWanda are good friends, and both are ADD. Both work as sales representatives in the women's fashion industry. Both enjoy what they do, are successful, and wish to stay in this line of work, but the similarity ends there.

Jamie's boss responds to her requests to make modifications because of her hypersensitivity. During most of the year, her boss lets Jamie set her own work hours, which allows Jamie to do paperwork in a quiet environment before others arrive at the office. This way, Jamie's sensitivity to noise and the action around her doesn't make her inefficient.

Jamie's boss also assigns an assistant to her when market is on, knowing Jamie will need time to get away from the noisy, stimulating environment. Jamie's sensitivity to other people's energy gets her overstimulated at these times, and having the assistant frees her to take a walk so she can clear her mind, collect her thoughts, and plan what she wants her next move to be. After twenty minutes off, she returns to the selling arena able to use her wonderful sales skills in an orderly way.

In contrast, LaWanda's boss knows only one way of doing things and neither understands nor wants to learn about alternatives. Everyone must come in at the same time and work in the same way. Though very good at what she does, LaWanda is miserable on her job and feels stressed and trapped much of the time. Though able to throw off the effects of the stress sometimes, she has begun to notice that she is getting more colds than usual and is developing a negative attitude about her work.

Though LaWanda blamed herself in the beginning, thinking she just wasn't doing enough, her friend Jamie pointed out some of the differences between their bosses. LaWanda is beginning to realize she may not be causing her problems by herself. Rather, her boss has to take some of the responsibility, even though it is LaWanda's hypersensitivity that creates the need for adjustments.

When LaWanda tried to talk to her boss about what she needs to feel better, he said he couldn't make an exception or everyone would want something different. So, LaWanda is considering trying to get on with another company—maybe Jamie's.

Job Evaluations: A Boss's Business

The annual ritual of evaluation provides a wonderful example of the effects of hypersensitivity and highlights ways a boss can make your life horrible or better. Your boss's job comes with the responsibility to perform the chore. Just as the boss can misuse other forms of power, this, too, can be used as a weapon.

Though no one enjoys being evaluated on the job, people with ADD feel the experience especially keenly. However, assuming that evaluations are looked at as a means to guide both job performance and professional growth, they can become positive guidelines for you. To the degree to which you are able to be self-aware and self-directed, your evaluation of yourself on the job can be used in partnership with your boss's insights.

To overcome the effects of your sensitivity, I'd strongly recommend that you speak with your boss ahead of time about the criteria upon which you are to be evaluated. Though primarily self-employed, I did this with one boss I had in the radio business. Because of my hypersensitivity, I asked that he tell me what he did want me to do rather than what he didn't want me to do. I reassured him that my intent was to please him and that I couldn't do it by finding out what was wrong. I could do it, or would ask him how to do it, when I knew what was wanted. I've never found any other approach that made sense to me.

Because of your hypersensitivity, you may feel torn up inside by criticism. That is not useful for anyone. Depending upon the type of ADD you have, you may find yourself responding by talking about the "stupid company" or "stupid boss," blaming everyone and everything around. On the other hand, you may blame yourself, feel guilty, and become depressed "because of the poor job" you are doing.

Please remember that everyone does the very best that he can at a given moment. You do, too. When you know a better way to accomplish something, you'll do it that way. Your boss may not know a better way to handle evaluations, yet he may be open to learning how to most effectively perform his function with you. Take your courage in hand and be open with him about your sensitivity, unless you judge that he or she cannot be understanding or flexible or will hurt you further.

Taking Things Personally

A.J. sells soft drinks to large chains. One day after he'd been out marketing a particular promotion, he returned to headquarters to discover his boss had made a change in the pricing structure of the deal. However, his boss had neglected to tell him of the change, so A.J. had made sales based on incorrect numbers.

Instead of realizing that the boss made a mistake, A.J., who is ADD, immediately saw the whole situation as his fault. "I must have missed what was being said in a sales meeting," he thought. "There I go again: I keep screwing up. I'm such a failure." His thoughts ran rampant, he felt miserably guilty.

He was afraid to go to his boss to clear the whole thing up. He was afraid to go to the customers and try to renegotiate the deals. He didn't know what to do.

Then he questioned the bond of trust he'd previously had with his boss, so he began to avoid looking his boss in the eye or even going near him. It wasn't until another employee complained about the boss's mistake that A.J. realized he'd reacted to a mistake that wasn't his own.

From his point of view, the boss didn't have a clue what was going on with A.J. All he sensed was a change in A.J.'s behavior, which made him nervous, worried, and irritable. The boss began to discount A.J., thinking he didn't know what he was doing. Really, all he was picking up was A.J.'s outward response to taking the blame to heart.

One or two incidents where your hypersensitivity shows won't cause too much trouble. When your boss begins to feel as if he or she must walk around on eggshells, however, tension is likely to build. Ultimately, though it would be very good if your boss would be the one to change, he or she doesn't need to—you do, as the employee.

Impulsivity

Acting and speaking without thinking can get you into a lot of trouble on the job. Even jumping to conclusions is a form of impulsivity; mentally failing to take the time to think before you really know what is going on can lead to faulty conclusions. People with ADD often have trouble in more than one area of impulsivity. Those around you tend to expect more from you than you can deliver, thinking that you ought to be able to engage your brain before you do, say, or think something. When you don't, you're likely to be called a child.

You're not a child. It's just that your neurochemistry does not give you the help that is offered to other adults as they mature. You have matured, too, but you must also learn to overcome the effects of being impulsive, which stems not from faulty learning or maturation, but from the way you're wired.

A.J. impulsively jumped to the conclusion that it was he who was at fault for not catching the pricing change. Carroll's impulsivity in response to the same situation showed itself differently. He was also caught by the boss's error, but unlike A.J., Carroll shoots off his mouth before he even begins to think through what he might want to say. Impulsively, Carroll stormed into the boss's office and yelled, "What the hell is going on here? I spent all day working my tail off, and you changed the pricing without telling me."

Now Carroll didn't yet know that, in fact, he was right and the boss had changed the pricing. He *assumed* it was the boss's fault. Again, though, the issue isn't whether the boss did or didn't change it without telling anyone. The issue is the way in which Carroll reacted to the situation with his boss. Telling a boss off, generally, is not the better part of wisdom, especially when an innocent mistake has been made.

Temper

To be sure, people with ADD often make very good salespeople. When the boss messes up by not passing up-to-date information along, those sales as well as the reputation of the salesperson are jeopardized. Again, sensitivity enters the picture, and the person with ADD will tend to take the loss of sales and reputation personally.

Blowing up doesn't help. Many people with ADD are prone to have "healthy" tempers. Like impulsivity, temper outbursts are often the result of a sensitive person's experiencing a threat, real or perceived, stress, or lack of support. Still, blowing up at the boss is not a good idea. Fortunately, both impulsivity and temper can be managed with training.

Taming Impulsivity and Temper

Hypersensitivity in a person with ADD contributes to the way he or she handles stress. Overreactions occur frequently, though when you factor in how sensitive the person is, the reaction is actually appropriate.

The way in which the reaction expressed, however, may need work. Quitting, mouthing off, or crucifying yourself are reactions that are not constructive, for yourself or anyone else. It's your job to get control of your hypersensitivity, impulsivity, and temper.

You can do it with training. Become aware of the kinds of situations that set you off. Notice if a certain kind of boss makes you feel better or worse. Ask yourself how much support you need in order to feel good on the job. Then ask whether it is reasonable for you to expect to get that much from your boss.

Ask yourself the following questions: Does your boss or his authority remind you of one of your parents? Did your parents or someone else hurt you with their authority? Were you made to feel guilty? Do you feel that your boss should protect you, fix things for you, hurt you, or be against you?

After you've considered these questions, you can begin to sort out the differences between your childhood experiences and those in the workplace. Then you can tell yourself on the job, This is not home; I am not a child. I have other ways to deal with the situation.

To live in peace with your boss, you must commit to change the way you respond in stressful situations. You can break the habit of automatically responding with hurt to difficult work situations. Be prepared to protect yourself in other ways than losing your temper, running away, or blaming your boss.

Do whatever it takes to get in the habit of stopping before you erupt. Put a reminder on your desk that says, "Stop and think before I act."

When your boss calls you in for a meeting, say to yourself, No matter what he says, I will ask questions before jumping to conclusions and think before I act.

If you have recently lost your temper with your boss, go back tomorrow and say, "I lost my temper with you last week. I am working on not doing that, because I know that it is not a good idea. I would appreciate it if you would accept my apology."

Then ask your boss to help you. This is assuming that the person is at least somewhat mentally healthy and willing to work with employees. You could say, "You could help me by telling me something good before telling me what I did wrong" or "When you change you mind about something, I would be able to deal with it better if you would let me know before I went out on the road." A great question to ask your boss, or anyone else for that matter, is, "Did you mean to hurt me when you said . . . ?" Often the person asked is aghast, not having any idea that you might be hurt. Their intent was totally different.

When Calvin failed to ask Marvin, his chief mechanic, to accompany him to a citywide trade show, Marvin felt slighted. They'd always had a good relationship, so Marvin decided to ask whether Calvin had intended to hurt his feelings. Amazed, Calvin said, "No. I didn't ask you because I thought you were all backed up with work and would be irritated about having to take time out for the show. I didn't mean to leave you out."

Some bosses ought not be in an authority role because they don't know how to handle power. Others aren't particularly well trained to manage people. Not all bosses, though, are the "bad guys." If you have a problem with all the bosses you work for, you would probably benefit either from doing some soul searching about yourself or from counseling about why this is the case. You'll feel a lot better when you get this problem under control.

When Your Boss Is Always Wrong and You're Always Right

If everything your boss does and says seems wrong to you, it's just possible that you are in an adversarial relationship with authority figures. If your boss says something is black and you say, "No, it's white," you fit the label *oppositional*. Oppositional behavior means that no matter what the other person says or does, you take the opposite position or go against the person's desire.

Children who say no consistently, do the opposite of what parents or teachers desire, or argue at the drop of a hat have been called Oppositional-Defiant for some years. They are frequently accused of being insensitive.

I have come to understand them in a new light. I have observed that such children, usually acquiring these labels in the early school years, tend to be quite active and verbal and have a mind of their own. Just the opposite of their negative assessment is true: they are actually *very* sensitive; so much so that they must fight to push away all the hurtful things that happen to them, things they experience as abuse. What are being described here are Outwardly Directed ADD children who are hypersensitive and express emotions and behavior emphatically and loudly.

What has been missed in the past are the incidents that preceded the "opposition." These incidents begin to occur immediately at birth, with the painful intrusions of light, sounds, injections, and the like. By school age the resistance to such intrusions has become habit, even when there may be no actual threat. By adulthood the habit is even more established. It always was and continues to be an attempt at self-protection.

In the workplace, where power lies in the hands of authority, bosses often trigger remembrance of all the times when the person was hurt, though perhaps unwittingly, by authorities: parents, teachers, coaches, and other adults. The more a child was taught, "I'm the authority. Do this because I tell you," and "I will make you," the bigger the problem will be in adulthood.

When Cary, a salaried employee, received a memo from his boss stating that time clocks were to be installed, he bristled and immediately determined that he'd have no part of them. No one could make him punch in and out—no one was going to have that kind of control over him. He was considering quitting his job because of it.

What Cary didn't realize was that the time clocks were the cheapest way to keep track of workers' actual hours, making sure they could get their proper shares of year-end bonuses. Overtime beyond expected salaried hours was to be factored into bonuses. The time clocks were actually for Cary's benefit.

Cary never asked. He automatically resisted anyone's having any control over him. It made him feel trapped, intruded upon, and disrespected, yet neither his boss nor the company management intended it that way.

Cary demonstrated a reaction that he'd developed to protect himself for as long as he could remember. His mother was very controlling, possibly with Highly Structured ADD, and was always demanding things of him. She didn't know how to negotiate and forced him to do things her way. For as long as he could remember, everyone was forcing him to do things that he didn't want to do or that were not very good for him. He *had* to protect himself.

Cary's boss thought Cary was an uncooperative employee. He was fed up with Cary fighting him at every turn, especially since he tried to do things to make the lives of his employees better. He just didn't understand Cary, and, frankly, he was sick of putting up with him.

If Cary's boss were to get fed up enough, he would begin considering the possibility of letting Cary go. The first opportunity to cut staff back could easily become the opportunity he was looking for to get rid of a particular "troublemaker." After all, bosses don't like their jobs to be too hard any more than workers do.

It is not the boss's responsibility to ask what lies under the oppositional behavior demonstrated by Cary. If he had never been exposed to the concept, he wouldn't even suspect that there was a sensitive, hurt part of Cary that actually needed his protection. For his part, Cary is doing nothing to teach his boss what he really needs. He's just reacting.

When any of us experiences anger and oppositional behavior coming at us, we tend fight back. Even if I know what lies under it, my first reaction is to self-protect. Only later do I remember, "Oh, this means the person is frightened." When I was a psychotherapist seeing a client, I was always on guard for this kind of behavior. Outside the walls of the highly controlled therapeutic environment, no one is going to watch that carefully. The workplace is not a therapeutic setting.

What Can Be Done?

It's up to Cary to recognize how he reacts. He needs to know that very real reasons initially existed for his defensiveness. He actually did a very good job trying to protect himself, even if his behavior was not understood that way by the people around him. He needs to be commended for being so responsible.

However, he also has to recognize that his reaction has become a habit. Now, as an adult, he has the words to ask what others mean when they do or say something that frightens him. Yes, he must realize that he is actually frightened, and he must use his words to find out whether there is any reason to be frightened.

He could ask to speak to his boss or personnel department so he could ask why a time clock system was being installed, rather than jumping to a conclusion. Then, if he still felt bad about having to use it, he could ask if there were some other way he could keep track of his hours. Otherwise, would his boss or another worker be willing to help him clock in and out so it wouldn't feel so bad?

Maybe he'll even be afraid that he'll forget and then get cheated. A buddy system could help him in this instance. With openness and honesty about what he feels, armed with understanding the self-protective purpose of his alarm system, and knowing he can get help with mastering the change, Cary could get the relief he needs, while his employer can get what is needed for the job.

Previewing Your Boss: What to Look for during a Job Interview

A lot of problems on the job can be avoided if you place yourself in the right environment in the first place. When interviewing for a job, it is important that you have, or quickly get, a good feeling about the person who is going to be your boss. Though I know this is hard when you need work, you could be jumping from the frying pan into the fire if you take a job with a boss who you don't feel very good about.

Harry had been out of work for some time. Not only was he running short of money, but his self-esteem was suffering. A friend told him about a job nearby. During the interview, he really didn't much like the man who ran the company, but he figured he could ignore his feelings and just do the job.

Wrong! Without respect for his boss, Harry quickly found himself in worse trouble. His boss didn't seem to much like Harry, either, and had hired him because his friend had put a good word in for him. The boss's displeasure of having hired someone he didn't much like caused him to ride Harry constantly. Harry continually made faces when the boss asked him to do something. That only made the boss more irritable, until he fired Harry one day.

By this time, Harry was so depressed that he felt he'd never be able to work again. After all, he hadn't been able to get work for a long time, and when he finally did, he couldn't keep the job. His conclusion: he must really be useless and unemployable.

Finding the Right Boss for You

To find the right boss, you need to become aware of your specific type of ADD. Go back to pages 8–9. Figure out what type or types of ADD you are. Then go to pages 110–114 to see what type of boss is best suited to you.

Make a list of the characteristics that you feel you would like to have in a boss. Be as complete as you can. Then, when you interview for a job, even a temporary one, look for those characteristics. Be careful that the person interviewing you is actually the one with whom you'll be working. I've had situations when a higher-level boss and I got along very well, only to discover later that my immediate supervisor and I did not share the same philosophies or work styles. The results were not pleasant.

Most important, during the interview listen to your intuition, which tells you whether you feel comfortable with the person. Be cautious that you don't try to talk yourself into respecting someone whom you don't respect. And don't assume that just because someone is in a supervisory role, he or she knows how to manage people.

Remember to be aware of whether the person has as much emotional power as job power. Ask yourself whether the person has at least as much or more emotional power than you. Ask yourself whether you can learn from this person.

Be clear about what you want your boss to do for you. Too many people spend all their interview time trying to sell the boss on themselves, rather than also interviewing the boss to see whether the situation is a good fit.

You might ask what the prospective boss expects from you. Ask what the person wants to accomplish—the goals that you would be a part of meeting. This can vary anywhere from getting twenty reports out of the typing pool a day to building a concert hall. The goal may be to increase sales by twenty percent or to dig safer trenches at a construction site.

Next ask what is expected from you. "How do I fit into your picture? What do you need me to do to accomplish the job you want done?" If you have ideas, different from those the boss has expressed, that might contribute to reaching that goal, suggest one and see how the boss responds. If he discounts it or seems to not want to be bothered, you know he's not open to options and probably isn't very flexible. If that's okay with you, then fine. If you want to be a more active participant in the planning and development of your role, then it probably wouldn't be a very good setting for you.

Get a reading on the boss's personality. Does he seem sensitive, calm, excitable, brusque, or all business? Do you like the kind of person you're talking with? Do you feel compatible? Would you like to get to know him better? Do you feel respect for him?

Does the boss to respond to the kind of person you are? Notice whether he responds to your humor. Does he nod when you get excited about something about the job he's telling you? Does he ask your opinion? Is it important to you that he care?

Do you seem to be able to understand one another, or do you continually have to ask questions to get the meaning of what each other is saying? In particular, does he ask questions of you in order to understand you? If your boss is a very linear thinker, paying attention to detail and being quite concrete, whereas you are a creative person who gets all excited about the overview of a situation, you are likely to have trouble communicating. That is not a reason to not work together, but it will have to be worked with. In fact, part of the interview could consist of acknowledging the value of each other's talents and skills while committing to work on bridging the differences.

Try to determine how organized your boss is and how organized he expects you to be. Ask what kinds of help are available to assist you, if organization is difficult for you. Get a clear picture of support staff availability for you, if you're interviewing for that kind of job.

Notice how perfectionistic your boss is and compare it to how perfectionistic you are or want to be. Are you willing to work within his limits? I recall one airplane mechanic who quit his job because he was working for a boss who did not have high standards of mechanical excellence in his shop: "Just get the job done and the plane back in the air." The mechanic had very high standards for his workmanship, feeling responsible for the safety of the passengers. He meticulously checked and rechecked his work to be sure the plane was safe, but his boss didn't want him spending so much time on each individual job.

When he interviewed for his next job, the aircraft mechanic specifically interviewed his potential boss about quality standards and presented a scenario that told him how his boss-to-be and the company felt about quality. He was pleased and took the job, and he has been quite satisfied.

Check on the boss's flexibility toward working with your differences. You may or may not decide to say you are ADD, but either way, you can check on his attitude about flex time, mobility, and willingness to work with your creativity. If you need to be out of the office a lot, would you be allowed to do your expense reports at home? How demanding is the boss about reflecting the corporate image versus letting your individuality show? Would you have opportunities to let your creative thinking develop?

One computer programmer cut a deal with a potential boss to do the company's work eighty percent of the time, while being allowed to develop creative programs for the company's use the other twenty percent of the time. He found out that this would be possible during the interview process.

Harriet, with school-age children, asked during interviews whether she could get someone to cover for her when special school events came up during the day. She would be responsible for getting someone to cover her shift, as long as her boss approved of her doing it. She turned two jobs down before finding a boss who would work with her. They have now worked satisfactorily together for several years.

Changing Bosses in the Company

Obviously, the boss you hire under may or may not stay as long as you do, or you may have the opportunity to get promoted to work for someone else. Transitional times when bosses change can be very stressful, but consider a change in boss much like the initial interview. If the boss doesn't have each employee come in for a meeting, ask for one to get acquainted.

Though you don't have to make snap judgments, check the person out and listen to your own inner feelings. Be aware that everyone runs her job uniquely. Your new boss may do things that please you and be willing to work with you, but he may not. Just because you are working for the same company does not mean that you will always be treated the same way. Be aware that you have options.

In summary, recognize the power that a boss has in relation to you. Know your needs. Assess what you can and want to change about yourself, and what you can't or don't want to. Finally, know what you want out of a boss and go get it. A boss-employee match is available for everyone, only it may take time to find it.

7

Stress on the Job

L et's suppose you work for a retail store that is expanding into a superstore to be opened in eight days. As a department manager, you are responsible for readying the old merchandise and giving the OK for items that will be added to the new store's stock. You've worked fourteen days in a row with no break. Your wife, whose schedule has also been heavy, is tired and angry, too. Your kids miss you. When you get to work in the morning, the clerks are lined up with questions. Customers can't find what they're looking for. To top it all off, you think you're coming down with a virus.

Sound familiar? Though you may never have worked as a retail sales manager, you can probably empathize and imagine the stress of this employee. In this chapter I'm going to discuss stress, so that you can learn which stress issues everyone faces, and which ones are particular to people who are ADD.

The average stress that everyone else feels is magnified by your hypersensitivity if you are ADD. The areas in which your ADD creates difficulties will probably cause you more stress than your non-ADD counterpart—for example, feeling harried when you are trying to get organized. However, you must remember that everyone has strengths and vulnerabilities. What you do easily, your counterpart may have trouble accomplishing. Know that stress is a part of everyone's life; it's just that yours belongs to you and causes you the trouble. So let's look at particular areas that are likely to concern you.

The Job Stressors We All Know

Stressors are the situations, relationships, and job demands that make us feel stressed. We all have some, but what causes stress for one person might not cause stress for another. Let's take a look at some of the more common stressors—ones that you're probably all too familiar with.

The first job stressor has to do with job fit, that is, how well you fit the job in which you find yourself. Maybe you took your current job because you needed the income, but you knew it wasn't really going to be the right job for you. Many of us find ourselves in this situation more than once in our lives. It's one of the ways we learn about ourselves, but it can be a painful lesson—one that needs to be learned quickly, then left behind.

I remember spending three awful, horrible, painful months as the director-manager of a day-care center. Though I knew a lot about children and good programming, I didn't have a clue how to deal with the management and administration of the center. Making decisions about how much food to order, payroll taxes, and the city health department were nightmares for me. I was a total failure, and finding out how much of a failure I was created enough stress for me to get sick on the job, a rarity for me. I have rarely been so glad to turn in my resignation. I'm guessing that it was not a moment too soon—or I'd have been fired. I should have been fired. From that experience I learned I am no administrator of anything.

Everett, a lawyer because his dad was one, was taught that being a lawyer was a "good way to earn a living." Actually, Everett was artistically inclined and dreamed of a career as an artist and set designer, but he never told anyone. He figured he'd become involved with community theater after he was established in his law practice. Ten years later, however, he was still working overtime to keep up at work and was too depressed and apathetic to do anything else.

Being in a job that doesn't fit you, or in a job that you don't like, creates a mountain of stress which is likely to turn into physical or emotional problems, such as depression.

If you've ever found yourself working with people you don't much like, you know the meaning of stress. Rest assured it probably won't get much better. The stress of spending time daily with people you don't get along with leaves its marks. Think about the people you work with and for, and ask yourself how you feel when you're with them.

Try this interesting exercise: Draw a small circle, representing yourself. Then around that small circle, draw more small circles, representing all the people with whom you work. Label each with the name of the person. Next, put a plus, minus, or zero sign by each small circle representing whether the person adds to your well-being, takes away from it, or has no effect on you one way or the other.

You will tend to feel stressed with each person you've marked with a minus sign. You'll feel enriched by each one with a plus sign. Now add the minuses and pluses to see what your overall sum is. This will tell you whether you're running a deficit account in the workplace or coming out ahead people-wise, even though there may be some other stresses.

You cannot continue to work indefinitely with more minuses than pluses, or you will begin to see an erosion of your mental and physical health. But you're not helpless. Though other persons may be the sources of stress, it's your responsibility to do something about it in order to protect your health and well-being.

Difficulties between people at work are often called "personality conflicts." What this usually means is that other persons reflect a part of you that you don't want to look at. Otherwise, it could mean that they are so different, you don't understand them, and their ways make you uncomfortable, especially if they try to assign their way of doing things to you.

Mandy saw a reflection of herself in her coworker Laura. Laura tended to be a critical, judgmental woman who talked about people behind their backs. Mandy hated those characteristics, but on deeper review, she realized that she was judging Laura. Then Mandy became aware that she herself was critical, a characteristic that was itself a result of the way she was raised, and that she actually had very little sympathy for herself when she made a mistake. Mandy was seeing the critical aspect of herself reflected back to her by Laura's behavior, and it made her extremely uncomfortable.

Kramer disliked Fred for a different reason. The easygoing manner that endeared Kramer to his coworkers appeared in distinct contrast to the methodical, keep-everything-under-control approach taken by Fred. They cosponsored a seminar to provide continuing-education credits for mental health professionals. And they made each other crazy.

When it was over, Fred said he'd never work on any project with Kramer again, and Kramer felt relieved. Fred had wanted everything done ahead of time, planned and plotted out. Kramer needed to get a brief overview of the intent of the training, then spontaneously breeze in at the last minute and perform. Both did good presentation jobs, but they couldn't stand to work together.

Neither was "at fault," but both were stressed. Not working together again was a great idea for these two.

One of the biggest stresses known to humankind is the task of working while raising children. Single parents have it the worst. Both physically and emotionally, the strain creates fatigue, anxiety, worry, and depression as well as poor work production.

Physically, there is never enough time in the day to do everything that needs doing. Rushing to pick up the children cuts into time needed for work. Trying to decide what to do and how to do it creates stress when a child is sick, needs a ride somewhere, or has a school performance that the parent doesn't want to miss.

Emotional stress comes when you are worried because your child is having trouble in school, the siblings aren't getting along, or one summer morning you're asked, "Daddy, why do I have to go to day care? Why can't I stay home like other kids?" Talk about being distracted!

A troubled marriage, visits from difficult in-laws, money problems, and even the neighbor's dog digging in your garden all create distractions because of the stress they generate. Also, keeping secrets from your coworkers adds tension—secrets such as the affair you're having or your husband's drinking problem. Maybe your husband is being transferred, and you can't tell anyone. Or maybe you are in an abusive relationship, and you're too ashamed to let anyone know.

To these problems, add health problems that are very wearing—either short-term or long-term—especially if you're afraid your boss or coworkers will think you might not be able to do your job well because of them. Maybe you're just plain frightened about your physical health. Maybe you had an auto accident, and your insurance might be canceled.

As you already know, the list of stressors just goes on and on and on.

Everyone has stress some of the time, but some people seem wed to stress all the time. If crisis has become a way of life for you, then it's time to seek help to break the cycle. If the situation has reached that point, then, like it or not, you are unintentionally contributing to the creation of the crisis.

On the other hand, there are times in your personal life when stress is on the increase only temporarily. Times of transition—during a move, after a marriage or a divorce, when you become a parent, or when children leave home—produce normal feelings of stress. Losses of all kinds create normal stress also, and during those times you need to go easy with yourself.

Usually, it's a good idea to tell your supervisor about such stresses. For a time, you can expect some support and understanding. Maybe your coworkers will help out by lightening your work load. You can expect to take at least six months to recover enough from most situations to become fairly functional again on your job. You may not be functioning at one hundred percent, because it takes a couple of years to completely overcome major losses and stress, but you'll be able to carry your part of the load again.

If after six months you still feel unable to do your part, you'll need to consider renegotiating your job. Perhaps you can switch to part time or take a leave of absence. Talk with your boss about options.

Work load is another major job stressor. These days, with the downsizing of so many companies, it's not uncommon for one worker to be asked to do the work that was formerly shared with another or even more than one other. Sometimes you can reduce this kind of stress by working smart, but sometimes your boss has unrealistic expectations that no one can meet. Feeling as if you'll never see an end to the work makes depression a likely result.

It's important to talk with your boss after you have figured out how much work you can reasonably do and what you cannot do. Suggest other ways the work can be completed. Also, think through ahead of time what you will do if your boss doesn't want to listen or if her hands are tied and no relief is in sight.

If your boss is reasonable but can't change the work load, at least knowing that she understands and wants to help might help alleviate some of your stress. Together you might plan a "mental health day" every now and again, when you can take artificial breaks from the stressful situation. If your boss is unreasonable, you might want to take those days off anyway and just don't tell her. After all, stress sickness is just as good a reason to call in sick as having the flu. If you don't take the day off and get some relief from the stress you're feeling, you'll probably get the flu anyway.

We all have work areas in which we feel, and truly are, inadequate. When our job demands that we perform in these areas, stress is the result. Every month when I have to do my accounting—mind you, I do only enough to send something reasonable to my accountant—my head hurts after about ten minutes. It feels as if someone is tightening a vice around my forehead. Not a good feeling!

A doctor friend of mine gets stressed when he has to meet people socially. A fine diagnostician who knows all about his specialty, he rarely says a word outside of the office unless it's about medicine. He says he has always felt totally inadequate making small talk and has tried to overcome this feeling, but he feels so stressed that it's not worth the effort.

Another acquaintance of mine has no sense of direction. Anytime her job requires her to travel to a new location—and as a social worker, that is frequently—she frets, writes copious notes, and tries to get someone to drive there with her the day before so she can practice the route. I personally watched her face become colorless when she thought she was lost. Panic was not far behind. That's stress!

If you must bump into your area of weakness regularly on the job, it is a good idea to try to find some way to get around it. Teaming is one way. Being forthright with your boss is another. Perhaps someone else can be given the chore that stresses you.

A number of years ago, a skilled clinician on my staff experienced such high stress about being on my radio show that she vomited and was unable to go on. Normally very disciplined and adequate, she simply could not face the microphone. Though I felt she would be an asset to the show, I found someone else, needless to say, and in no way penalized her because of her vulnerability. We just worked around it.

If you are not performing up to the expectations of your job, you know it, and you also are going to feel enormous stress at work. This could have happened because you took a job that was beyond your skill level, or maybe the job turned out to be something different from what you thought it would be.

Of course, you might not be meeting job expectations because of outside distractions. Then it's up to you to be honest with yourself and your coworkers. By taking responsibility for your lack of performance, you and others can make accommodations.

Sometimes, however, your inability to perform is not your fault at all. For example, consider Roy. Roy took a job as a media writer-publicist for a politician who was positioning himself for re-election. Roy was good at his work. However, he soon discovered that the politician and her assistant were on two different tracks and were accomplishing nothing. Roy couldn't get them to identify their goals and stick with them. Roy had no power on the job to set goals, so he was helpless to do his job. As a result, he began to question his worth and skills.

The most common reason people cannot meet job expectations is that they are given responsibility without the power to implement whatever needs to be done. This is a no-win situation. With the help of a consultant, the lines of responsibility can occasionally be ironed out. If not, you'd better begin to cover your backside and figure out a way to get out before you are scapegoated for other people's inadequacies.

ADD: Compounding Stress on the Job

There is one underlying issue that compounds the problem of job stress for people with ADD, and it is this: they already have so many other stressors in their lives, they just don't have room for more. I'm sure you know what I mean when I talk about an accumulation of stress because of ADD, especially if your ADD went undiagnosed or untreated most of your life. Because you were continually expected to have skills that are difficult for you, and because your way of doing things is different from that of the majority culture, you have probably endured high levels of stress, including from failure to reach your potential. I imagine that many of these stresses have been chronic, since you've been repeatedly expected to accomplish what is unnatural for you.

Consider Lawrence as a case in point. Lawrence is an engineer who learned his skills on the job. He has repeatedly been skipped over for promotions because he didn't have a college degree and hasn't been able to pass the professional engineering exam. However, Lawrence is so good at what he does that the college-trained engineers he works with come to him with the difficult problems they can't solve.

Never able to concentrate on written tests and book learning, he's failed the professional exam four times. Due to take it a fifth time, he found he just couldn't try any longer. He knew how to do his job, and his work was top notch, but taking tests was beyond him. So Lawrence quit his job, discouraged and experiencing many stress-related symptoms.

In some ways, we are much like a piece of elastic in clothing, which pops back into shape after it's stretched—at first. At first we recover quickly, too. However, a year later, after repeated stretching, the elastic no longer recovers; it might even break apart. Human emotions are much the same way. Stress accumulates unnoticed until one small event makes a person snap. It's the proverbial straw that breaks the camel's back.

The fact that a person has ADD predisposes her to be more vulnerable and possibly less likely to handle stress well. When additional stress, even normal stress, accumulates, the breaking point can come more quickly. Let's take a look at how this happens.

As we've discussed, people with ADD are hypersensitive to the physical attributes of the workplace, whether noises, smells, or the comfort of their chairs. For example, without having paid any direct attention to the fabric I'm sitting on, I can tell you whether I experience it as pleasant or intrusive. If I sense it as rough or slick, I have to make a mental adjustment to block out that feeling so that it doesn't distract me from my goal. Though one adjustment to your chair's surface in one day isn't much, taken together with all the other minute adjustments of the day, it adds up to a lot of distraction. The result is stress.

Maybe you find yourself thinking about the stress that comes from other people in the workplace. Being hypersensitive, not only are you disproportionately aware of what they are feeling, but you may also empathize with them. Both your awareness and your empathy can place you under stress.

Suppose your place of employment is getting ready to implement a major change. It hasn't been announced yet, but because you are hypersensitive, you begin to feel that something is amiss. You sense the tension but can't place where it's coming from. All you know is that you feel stressed, but you can't figure out why.

That happened to me when I was a radio talk show host in the early 1980s. Unbeknownst to the employees, management had made the decision to change from a talk format to a music format. The first any of us knew about the change was the Friday afternoon we were called in and given our pink slips.

To the surprise of many of my colleagues, I was not shocked. I actually felt relieved to know exactly what was happening, because I had felt that something was wrong for some time. The stress of not knowing *what* was wrong was much worse for me than discovering the cause of the tension. My experience is typical of people who have ADD. We know things ahead of time, even if we don't know exactly *what* it is that we know.

If you're hypersensitive, receiving criticism is a tremendous source of stress. In addition to the formal evaluation process that we discussed in the previous chapter, criticism of performance, dress, image, and even beliefs can run rampant in many work settings. Those critical words, even when gently communicated, can feel like a knife in the gut.

Have you ever walked away from a meeting feeling as though you'd been run over by a truck? Maybe all that happened was that your new design was not greeted with enthusiasm. Perhaps someone made a suggestion he thought might improve your design. As a result, your heart may have actually felt physically squeezed. Unless a person is hypersensitive, it's hard to image how much stress can be felt physically as well as emotionally, but the physical pain is present nevertheless.

If you remain silent after hearing criticism, it's bad enough. Some people with ADD fight back, that is, mouth off, compounding the situation and the stress. That creates a second layer of stress, as bosses and coworkers react to your explosion. This could be where the term double whammy came from, and you are the recipient of both punches. Pretty soon, you feel as if you'll never be able to reverse the buildup of stress.

The low self-esteem of people with ADD sets them up to have their worst fear, failure at work, realized. If you live with this fear, you probably feel you need to constantly prove yourself on the job, and that adds stress.

You also probably tend to interpret everything in negative ways, which makes the workplace more stressful than it really needs to be. For example, when Jeremy did not see his name on a list of employees who were to be moved to a new facility, he immediately assumed he was being let go because he wasn't good enough. He suffered greatly—until he found out that the ommission of his name was a clerical error.

Constant feelings of inadequacy can cloud your ability to see opportunities for advancement. Hiding from those who have the power to promote, in order to hide your inadequacies, means you are not showcasing your talent, playing office politics, and selling yourself to your superiors. You thus create the lack of advancement without realizing you are doing it. Then you feel stressed because your worst fears have come true.

Feeling like a loser makes you carry yourself like a loser. I remember a real estate agent, Teresa, whose posture was poor because she was always trying to hide in the background. As she moved, I could see and feel how little she thought of herself. The question immediately came to my mind, How can you sell my house for a good price when you don't feel good about yourself? As I hesitated, she slumped even more, eyes downcast, as if she'd expected me to reject her. Though my heart went out to her, I chose not to work with her.

She had obviously lost good feelings about herself at an earlier time and now was losing more of her self-esteem daily. She lost my business and an opportunity to begin a new career. She lost money, and she lost respect. These are a lot of losses. All of these are major stress producers.

Possibly the worst loss was that of her self-worth. While I was in the office, a colleague of hers could be overheard being praised for the fine job she'd done for an older couple buying a retirement home. My potential agent flinched as she heard the remarks and looked devastated as they sank in. Part of me again wanted to give Teresa my business to save her from her pain, but another part wasn't willing to risk financial loss for myself.

Patricia, a realtor more outgoing than Teresa, had a lot of trouble with the paperwork associated with sales. She was often not able to help customers secure financing which meant she, too, lost a lot of business. When other realtors in the office succeeded in making creative deals for their customers, she felt jealous and acted catty, talking behind their backs about doing things in "shady ways."

Predictably, and unfortunately for Patricia, this approach did not endear her to her colleagues. In fact, she created more stress than if she had been able to ask for help when she got stuck on a deal. Her jealousy gave her away. Patricia had very low self-esteem, which is always what underlies jealousy.

Dirk also has low self-esteem, but he shows his differently. As someone with Outwardly Expressive ADD, his extreme competitiveness gives him away. He can't stand to lose—anything. When he does, he experiences feelings he's long been trying to push far away. Sensitive beyond words, he never wants anyone to know how he really feels. So, no matter what the cost, Dirk must prove he is valuable, first to himself and then to everyone around.

Because so many people with ADD must work harder to accomplish the same task as a non-ADD counterpart, they wear themselves down mentally and physically. Fatigue, lack of balance in life, and fear of being left behind take their toll and create stress. In addition, keeping longer hours pulls people with ADD away from their families, which creates secondary stress.

"No one really understands," Philip said in his first training group for people with ADD. He'd been feeling so stressed—trying to get everything done and keep his family happy, too—that he started to tear up when he discovered that others did understand. "It's like being up against a wall and trying to beat it down, and it's so hard, and I can't do it. My wife tries to understand, but she can't. She wants to help, but I don't know what she can do. I have to do it, but I can't.

"My parents always said I should 'just do it.' For years I tried, but I couldn't 'just do it,' and they never believed me. Now I don't know if I believe myself. I think I should be able to."

Once these feelings of difficulty come, feelings of being overwhelmed are not far behind. They grab at Philip's throat. Next comes the feeling of inadequacy, then hopelessness and depression.

Sometimes on a job, if you work hard enough, you do finally "get it," but the price is high in terms of stress points. Take organization, for example. Once you've gotten into a groove with certain organizational tasks, you may be able to do them without so much stress and feel it's worthwhile to continue. Other times, you may decide, "No, I don't want to. I'll make a trade for this one. I'll find someone else to do this task for me, and I'll do something for her in return."

Most people with ADD recognize that there are times, though, when, no matter how hard you work, you're not going to get it. Balancing a logbook is a good example. If every time you try, you make a new or different mistake, you come to realize that there is an endless variety of potential mistakes that you can make—including remaking the ones you made earlier. Even if you total the right amount once, chances are you won't be able to total it again to verify that it's right. And that is very, very stressful.

By Philip's last meeting with his training group, he realized that if he couldn't get something done within a reasonable amount of time and effort, he needed to shift gears and team up with someone. "It's better for me to use my people skills to earn money and to hire someone to do the things I can't do well," he said.

I still find a lot of people with ADD who think that if they take enough medication, they might be able to do everything that is difficult, or impossible, for them now. They don't understand that's not the whole issue. Medication helps some people with some parts of their ADD, but it cannot change you into something you're not. If you and your doctor have decided that medication is appropriate for you, use it judiciously.

The Physical and Emotional Symptoms of Stress

When most people think about stress, they think about physical, mental, or emotional tension and strain. Usually stress is considered to come from the environment, other people, or events. Technically, any stimulus, such as fear or pain, that disturbs or interferes with the normal physiological equilibrium of an organism is labeled *stress*.

No one escapes stress. The more changes and, therefore, disequilibrium you experience, the more you are likely to feel stressed. As we have discussed, just having ADD begins the process of stress because of the lack of fit with the culture around you. Add to that the accumulation of stresses year after year through school, and now in the workplace, and you are likely to have what is called a *stress reaction*. To help you identify that reaction, use the following list of physical, mental, and emotional symptoms that tell you not only that stress is present, but that you need to begin to pay serious attention to it.

Because stress is now known to underlie many illnesses and other physical conditions, it is important to realize that once the body has begun to react to the stress by experiencing physical symptoms, they have taken on a life of their own and must be dealt with accordingly. If physical or mental symptoms of stress remain for more than a short period of time and are extreme or recurring, you need to see your doctor. It is better to find out that there is no cause for alarm than to miss an opportunity to help your body get healthy.

- **Headaches** frequently result from stress. You could experience tension that feels as if a band were being tightened around your forehead, or an ache at the back of your neck that radiates over your shoulders and between your shoulder blades, especially on the left side of your body. These are common stress-connected headache symptoms, but others are possible. Remember to check with your doctor if they recur or are severe, because there are many other reasons for headaches.

- **Other body aches and pains** also reflect stress. Often you will find that you've been holding a muscle rigidly, as if to ward off impending intrusion. As if to fight back, you clench your fist or your jaw.

- **Teeth grinding, nail biting, and hair twirling** can all be stress reactions. Although they can also be associated with other conditions, if they persist, you need to get them checked.

- **Many skin conditions** have a stress component that can be alleviated through stress reduction activities.

- **Illnesses such as heart problems and cancer** have been shown to have significant, though not exclusive, connections to stress. Certainly, such an illness can often be traced from the time it shows itself, back to a particularly stressful event or period.

- **Colds, viruses, and bacterial infections** can also frequently be traced to times of high stress. More than one person has become ill in the middle of a move or job change. "When it rains, it pours" is probably a stress-related saying. Sometimes these conditions strike as soon as a project is completed, during the letdown phase.

- **Accidents** occur much more commonly when people are under stress. Whether auto accidents or those in the home and workplace—falling off a ladder or stabbing yourself with a staple—during times of stress you are much more susceptible than others.

- **Fatigue and listlessness** indicate that your body, mind, and emotions are under pressure. Though these accompany many other physical problems, they are extremely common as reactions to stress.

- **Sleep difficulties** or changes also suggest the presence of stress. Of course, worrying can keep anyone awake.

- **Loss or increase of appetite** or any other major change in eating habits can also be a response to stress. Note when the change occurred and see whether it can be dated to a time of considerable stress. If other symptoms are present or last for any time, remember to check with your doctor.

- **Confusion**, or the feeling that your mind is filled with mush, is one of the most common feelings experienced with stress. When you feel overwhelmed and don't know what to do next, if you cannot think through a problem or situation like you used to be able to, you may feel this type of confusion. Remember, though, other reasons also exist for this feeling: reactions from hypoglycemia and related conditions, seizure disorders, and other brain-related conditions. If the symptoms continue, see a doctor.

- **Forgetfulness** rises rapidly under stress. You surely may, as someone with ADD, have had a lifelong problem with forgetting things, but under stress it becomes even worse. Know that you're in good company. Your mind may be on overload trying to manage more information or change than it can handle, so some of the information gets lost. That is due to stress.

- **Loss of mental acuity** occurs, too. Finding that you cannot think as quickly or precisely as you previously could is frightening. Maybe you just aren't as creative as you were previously. These can be the result of stress.

▪ **Disorganization** at a higher level than is normal for you may mean stress. Though already a characteristic of ADD, disorganization may indicate that you're under stress. Suddenly being less able than usual to keep track of things, losing your glasses or car keys more frequently, and having a greater difficulty keeping track of time are all common indicators of stress.

What you feel and how you feel about what is happening to you are indicators of stress in your life. Though such feelings may result from causes other than stress, ask yourself *when* they began, then check to see what was happening in your life at that time. Sometimes there is a delay before you experience the emotions connected to stress, so give yourself a window of a few weeks between the times changes or stressors occurred and symptoms followed.

▪ **Worry** is one of the most common responses people have to stress. In a way, it is the mind's attempt to figure something out to alleviate the stress. Though worry never solved anything, it can highlight a problem that needs your attention.

▪ **Depression** often covers the obvious presence of stress. Rather than being able to express your feelings openly, you may keep them inside. Saying, "Oh, everything is just fine," when in reality you feel that everything is falling down around your shoulders is the first sign that you are "stressed to the max." When you can't get out of bed in the morning, have lost your appetite, have become forgetful, feel as if life has no meaning, or feel trapped on an endless treadmill of life, you probably are depressed. Depression in this case is an emotional condition (as opposed to the biochemical), and it can be treated effectively with medication. There is no need to suffer.

▪ **Anxiety** that sort of drifts through you, not specifically attached to any one situation, may be coming from stress in your life. Often you are likely to feel it in the pit of your stomach, making eating unpleasant.

▪ **Panic attacks** are usually associated with stress, often accompanied by unrecognized anger. For someone already feeling out of control, the panic attack further exacerbates the feeling he or she is "going to die." Panic attacks sometimes make people feel as if they are having a heart attack. They may be accompanied by hyperventilation, which makes you unable to take in sufficient breath to breathe normally. Consult a physician if the condition does not pass quickly or you are in doubt. Help is available for panic attacks.

- **Obsessive and compulsive feelings** can result from stress, though either type can appear as full-fledged clinical conditions on its own. In response to stress, you may find yourself checking and rechecking whether you have your keys with you or have remembered to turn off the water. You probably will find that your mind is thinking about something else at these times, and that "something" is related to the stress you are feeling. You might discover that you want to make use of rituals that were never previously part of your life, such as putting your left shoe on before your right or sweeping the floor daily before you begin other activities. When this is a passing activity, lasting a few weeks at most, you can fairly well assume it's a reaction to stress. You're simply trying to get some order in your life, which turned chaotic on you. Once you reestablish order in your life, you'll find that you don't need these rituals anymore.

Remember, each of these symptoms could indicate that you are under stress, or it could be a part of a bigger picture requiring the assistance of a doctor or a counselor. No one, not even a professional, can tell initially whether you are having a stress reaction or that something else is occurring without an in-depth study. Even if you have a medical condition, stress may be a large component of what is going on with you.

Therefore, it is useful to be aware of the amount of stress you're under, do all you can to prevent its buildup, and use stress reduction techniques as needed. Even when a secondary physical or emotional problem has been triggered, you will mend better and faster if you also use stress reduction methods to help you recover.

Preventing Stress

Just because certain aspects of your work have always been stressful, don't assume they must continue that way. Look around you now for five things that create stress at work. You might think about something as simple as dull pencils. Sometimes the simplest thing can continually irritate you. Then do something about it, like buying an electric pencil sharpener.

Maybe the cause of your stress is a little more complicated than pencils, such as a shop worker who continually borrows one of your tools without returning it. In that case, you have several choices, including giving him his own tool as a present. Or you might have a talk with him, saying, "Look, at first I didn't mind you borrowing my tool, but now I need you to get your own." You can just make a statement—no frills or apologies, just a statement.

Of course, the stress could be more serious, and you need to head off the development of symptoms by doing something now. Even if your stress is caused by a major problem, such as being in the wrong job, today is as good a day as any to start a transition to something you would like better. Sure, it might mean going back to school, or perhaps you will have to move. Then again, maybe there is an opening in the company you're already working for that you haven't heard about, so talking to your boss might do the trick. Whatever it is, do something now.

Remember, just because you've always done things a certain way does not mean you have to continue to do them that way. Just because you don't know how to do something a new way doesn't mean you can't learn. Ask questions.

The first thing you need to do is become aware of what is bothering you. Next, come up with five things you can do to change each stressful situation. You may want to talk with someone else in order to brainstorm ideas. Then choose one of the five to act on. Finally, act.

You probably don't think twice about the merits of brushing your teeth regularly. You just do it because you know its importance in the maintenance of your health. Do you realize, however, that relaxing is just as important to your overall health and well-being? It's not just something to do *after* you've become stressed or tired.

Regular time spent relaxing takes some planning, though. Finding that time depends upon your priorities. I encourage you to do it, regularly.

Once you have set the time aside for relaxation, you must decide how you want to relax. Here are a few alternatives. Try different ideas to see what feels good for you or what is easy for you. Don't force yourself to do anything that is difficult or uncomfortable.

- **Sleep** is the most obvious way to relax, but it's important to ask yourself, Do I truly relax when I'm sleeping? Some of the signs that your sleep is not relaxing include waking up still feeling tired, dreaming fitfully, and tossing and turning—the covers on the bed will give you away. Grinding your teeth while you sleep or waking with tense muscles are other signs. However, a good night's sleep can certainly be relaxing.

- **A bath** can be useful as a relaxation technique. You may want to add a cup each of baking soda and Epsom salts to the water. Many holistic health practitioners recommend this for relieving stress, and I've found it to be quite useful.

- Getting a **full body massage** is one of the most relaxing experiences, at least in my opinion. If you choose to try this, remember that not all massage therapists work well for everyone. Trust your sensitivity to determine who is right for you. Some people with ADD do not tolerate massages well or for long. You may want a shortened version, so be sure to let the therapist know when you've had enough. I've found that a massage at least once a month by someone I trust who also does aromatherapy, mixing her own combinations of fragrant oils, makes all the difference in the world for me. Like every other form of relaxation, this is not for everyone, but you might want to give it a try if you never have.

- People with ADD who practice **meditation** or engage in some form of **self-hypnosis** regularly report staying more focused and centered. There are as many kinds and techniques as there are people dreaming them up. Again, not every technique works for everyone. For example, I've found that it is virtually impossible for many people with ADD to totally clear their minds. Anyone who teaches this form as the *best* or *ultimate* form of meditation does not have ADD. Instead, using guided imagery may be a good way for people with ADD to start meditating. Listening to a tape or taking a class can lead you to the relaxed state you are seeking.

- **Breathing exercises** of all kinds, including yoga breathing exercises, are extremely useful. If you do nothing more than take deep breaths while stopped at a traffic light, you will begin to notice a feeling of being refreshed. Learning a couple of breathing techniques that you practice daily for a minute or two quickly forms a habit that is available to use anytime—and is free.

Everyone benefits from a simple regimen of relaxation that they have made a habitual part of their daily living. Having ADD makes it essential that you learn to relax and do it regularly. Make it a high priority.

Recreation and physical activity are also important stress reducers. But physical activity and recreation are not always the same thing. If you play tennis just for fun, just to enjoy hitting the ball back and forth, that might be your form of recreation. If you are in a highly competitive league, though, that physical activity can bring its own stress with it— the exact opposite of what you are trying to accomplish in recreation and relaxation.

If you sit at a desk all week, almost any form of movement can help you reduce stress, which is what recreation is supposed to be about. Recreate means to change, redo, or resuscitate yourself, mentally, physically, emotionally, or spiritually. Whatever the usual mode you work in, you will find relief and rejuvenation through doing something different.

People with ADD tend to run low on endorphins, the "feel-good" chemicals released in the brain during physical exercise, so physical activity tends to have that extra stress reducing benefit for them. The runner's high is a perfect example of this. Though many of us will not go to that length to get the endorphins flowing, all physical exercise, even in moderation, biochemically helps those of us with ADD to reduce stress.

On the other hand, if you work in a job that requires intense physical labor, additional physical activity might not feel rejuvenating to you. You might find your recreation in watching television.

You're the best judge of what makes you feel revived. Trust yourself, but be careful. In our culture a lot of activities listed under the heading of "recreation" do not necessarily lead to relaxation. Picture the killer bridge game, a game that adds tension to your brain and every muscle in your body. What about the golf game in which the player breaks his club in a fit of temper? These don't seem very rejuvenating to me.

Recreation does not necessarily mean relaxation. Suppose you work in a job that is rather boring, and you seek excitement when you're not working. In that case, maybe engaging in a high risk sport, such as race car driving or skiing difficult slopes, would be rejuvenating. Maybe you are interested in challenging the records set in rock climbing or, in a different vein, playing the commodities market for the challenge and thrill of it. A certain amount of rejuvenation comes from these intense, challenging situations, if they are different from what you normally do. Just be sure that you make some time for quiet and relaxation along with the time for exuberant, faster-paced activities. The balance will help you alleviate stress.

If you are in a job you don't much like, you may take up a hobby that excites you and in which you can become quite absorbed. That will help you reduce stress in the short term. In the long term, however, you may need to go back to school to prepare for a different type of career, and you might find that you need to give up your hobby for a while during the transition. By keeping your end goal in mind, with the knowledge that you can return to your hobby after a specific length of time, you can tolerate the stress temporarily. You can do this because you *remember* the good feelings associated the hobby. That memory, for a while, will serve the purpose of providing you with recreation.

I know it sounds corny, but good eating habits are essential to keeping stress under control. Going to the drive-through at the nearest fast-food restaurant, picking up high-calorie, high-fat junk food, so you can eat it on the fly as you're driving to whatever is next in your life—that only adds to your stress level.

I'm talking about sitting down to eat something healthy on a regular basis. When was the last time you took a picnic to a park or ate by the side of a stream? Do you sit down at least once a day to a leisurely meal?

Next, check what you eat. I'm not talking about consuming rich, fancy foods. You need a balanced diet that includes fruits and vegetables, complex carbohydrates, and some protein source. Nothing exotic or terribly complicated is necessary. Balance is the key.

Many people with ADD tend to have really poor eating habits, and I don't want you to be one of them. It won't do for you to get all your food intake at one meal. Nor will you benefit from skipping meals so you can have something "forbidden" later. Balance, balance, balance!

If it's hard for you to put yourself on a schedule, maybe you can get a friend to help you, or take a class that helps you plan or eat out at healthy restaurants. There is more than one way to plan healthy meals.

My son with ADD solved his dietary challenges by developing the "Vat Method." Every few days he made a big pot of brown rice, another of beans, another of turkey chili, and still another of some mixed vegetables. Then he baked a couple of chickens cut in parts. He stored each food item in a big container, which we called a vat. In the morning he filled another container with food from each of the vats. Some days he alternated a can or two of tuna fish for the chicken. Sometimes he substituted wheat or spinach pasta, or a baked potato in the microwave, for the rice. He might pour a whole can of corn over his mix of the day. He heated this in the microwave, tightly sealed, and left for school, food in hand.

My son developed this method in high school while training to be an offensive lineman in football and has continued it through college. We noticed that he seemed to feel a lot better and was more focused when he ate his own cooking than when he tried to find food at school or elsewhere. He'd eat some of it during lunch and would snack on it several other times during the day which kept his energy balanced. And he has taught me to follow suit! It works well for us.

Though the research is not yet in on the effects of various foods on people with ADD, I've noticed that high-sugar and high-fat foods seem to cause trouble and stress. The proverbial cup of coffee is another mainstay of people with ADD. However, I've heard many reports of people being able to change from drinking twenty cups of coffee a day to maybe two after they start taking medication. Less craving for sugar seems to be present, as well.

Food allergies also seem common for people with ADD. Mood swings, nervousness, increased forgetfulness, and confusion are all symptoms of food allergies as well as stress. It stands to reason that cleaning up your diet, which in turn eliminates many of the symptoms common to allergies and ADD, is a good idea. Possibly the hypersensitivity so common in ADD contributes to the development of these allergies. It could be your body's way of telling you that something is amiss. Pay attention, and you'll feel better and function more effectively.

A final word of warning. Alcohol and drugs are not recommended to reduce stress. Often used by people with ADD "to get some relief," in the long run they increase stress. Instead of using alcohol or drugs, become involved in training and educational management of your ADD, and you'll be happy you did. Get on a regular schedule, treat your body well, and you will find your level of stress decrease.

Recovering from Stress

Whether you have ADD or not, there is a series of steps you need to go through when you have experienced stress. Whether the stress results from a sudden crisis or it has accumulated over a long period of time, you can feel reassured that by going through these five steps, you will recover.

When your stress has been long in building, you may find that it takes longer to undo its effects. Your body and mind have gotten in the habit of being stressed, and you must teach yourself to react differently in all kinds of situations, even those that are not actually stressful.

For example, consider Rachel. Rachel had worked for many years in the customer service department of a major store. Though very good at her work, she took on a lot of her customers' stress. She felt responsible for satisfying them, but she had little power to affect store policy. As a result, she eventually developed an itchy skin irritation that was diagnosed to be stress related.

Rachel and a good friend decided to go into business for themselves. As an owner of a specialty shop, she wanted her customers to be satisfied, and she had the power to see that they were. She discovered that any time a customer questioned her about a product, she began to itch. Now she could take care of the customer's needs, but it was as if her body didn't quite realize that. It took a couple of years before Rachel no longer had an itchy reaction to questions or complaints. Finally the symptoms went away, but it did take time.

Often it takes less time to get over a acute crisis situation because the body and mind have not gotten into the habit of reacting to the stress. The more stresses in a short period of time, the greater the accumulation of stress you will experience. When the snap comes, the final crisis may be less the issue than all of the little stresses that had piled up beforehand.

These different patterns of stress require varying amounts of time to recover from. Be patient and kind with your healing. You can feel confident that you will recover, but there will be ups and downs in the process. That's just how humans are. Here are the five steps to stress recovery:

Step 1. Put yourself in a nurturing situation and, as much as possible, avoid the situations that are putting demands on you. Call in your markers, so to speak, and let others take care of you. Ask for what you need. It's your turn to be taken care of. Forget about being independent, creative, or adventurous. This is your time to take, not give.

Step 2. As you begin to think clearly again, look at your values, in both your personal and your work lives. Ask yourself what is really important in life. Ask yourself what lessons you can learn from what's happened to you. After all, the stress only stopped your forward movement for a time. It has also given you time to reconsider the path you've been on. You may discover that your beliefs have changed greatly and your path needs to change, too; maybe your beliefs are generally the same as they've always been, but with modifications brought about because of the stress. Either way, you've been given a gift—the gift of learning about yourself. Use it!

Step 3. Redefine yourself in relation to your new beliefs and values. This includes the role or roles you've been playing in the work world. Who are you besides who you've been for the last so many months or years? This is the time when you can redesign your identity. You have the opportunity to figure out what is natural for you now. The answers you get may be different from what you've been doing on the job, or they may be similar, but with a fresh coat of paint applied.

Step 4. Now it's time to build any new skills that are necessary to make the transition back to health and recovery. This step has to do with *things*. You will feel an urge to experiment, to experience new things, to try out the untried, or perhaps to be adventurous. You may wish to take little steps initially. Your feelings will tell you how much to reach out. You may find that you'd like to try out some of your new skills under the direction of another person or situation. Just listen to your inner promptings and let yourself follow them. Do not listen to what others think you *should* do.

Step 5. The culmination of your recovery comes at this time. Your power is back in your own hands, and you can and need to do whatever supports the person you are now. You are no longer the person who was so stressed that you needed to regroup. You've gone through the process of self-discovery, and you've healed. You've reconsidered your values, updated your identity, and discovered and developed new skills or interests. Now it's time to put those interests and skills to work. Do it. The time is now.

You are recovered. You know how to ward off the accumulation of stress, and you know you can recover from stress. Whether you have ADD or not, you now have control and power over your life once again. You are wiser because of your experiences and can use them to make decisions at this time.

Applying these methods to the workplace, you no longer need to feel like a victim. Nor do you need to feel trapped. Given time, you can change whatever you want. By doing so, your job does not need to produce interminable stress in your life. Rather, it can showcase the person you are.

People with ADD: Creating Stress in the Workplace

Every coin has two sides. I'm sorry to have to tell you that those of us with ADD can create stress in the workplace, as well as experience it. All of the typical symptoms of ADD discussed in this book can create stress for our colleagues, coworkers, teammates, and bosses. Though we don't mean to be difficult, the truth is that we are not the easiest people to work with. Being honest about our limitations, though, and doing what we can to accommodate them will certainly help those with whom we work.

Hypersensitivity continues to create many problems for all concerned. Regardless of the type of ADD you have, your sensitivity will show; it just shows in different ways. It's no fun walking around on eggshells, which is what others often feel they have to do with us.

Organizational problems, too, are generic to ADD. The forms will vary by type, but you must become aware of how they affect others who don't know you are not just being lazy or irresponsible.

Your lack of concentration means that you might either be less effective than some of your coworkers or simply miss parts of what is going on. Again, your ADD hidden from view, your coworkers won't know whether you've just forgotten to follow through, you don't care to follow through, or you are a creative genius in outer space who doesn't think you should have to do the nitty-gritty work, which they must pick up.

Each type of ADD creates its own stress. People with Outwardly Expressive ADD can be "all over the place," rarely finishing anything. If you have this type of ADD, your timing may be grossly different from that of others who work with you. I have to watch this all the time. As far as I'm concerned, the minute an idea hits me, I figure it ought to be completely manifested and finished, leaving time for the next idea to burst forth for my attention. Needless to say, those who work with me are not totally comfortable, as they will still be trying to sweep up residue left from the first idea, while I've already gone on to the next project or adventure.

The creation of chaos is the offshoot of people with Outwardly Expressive ADD. Although well-meaning, you may find others getting mad with you. They may otherwise scold you for being irresponsible or scattered, which only means they are very, very frustrated trying to keep track of you.

People with Inwardly Directed ADD often seem not to be team players, off in the ozone of creative ideas or immersed in the intricacies of the project at hand. If you have this type of ADD and utilize your ability to empathize and help people, you may be trying to save the world, one person at a time. On a project, you can become so personally involved that a lot of time goes by while others are simply trying to get something—anything—done. You're also subject to burnout from wanting to adopt every child or person you meet, for example, rather than guiding them through the system, inadequate as it may be.

If you are Highly Structured ADD, your tendency to be controlling and perfectionistic can make others feel very uptight around you. You tend to lower morale in the workplace, undermining the effectiveness of teamwork and ultimately reducing productivity. You don't mean harm any more than the people with the other types of ADD do. After all, you're just trying to get a job done in the best way you know how. Yet, you must realize your way may not be the only way.

What can each of us do to alleviate the stress we create? First, recognize that you must take responsibility for your ADD. No federal legislation can demand that others accommodate you if you don't or can't take a responsible, active part in doing all you can do. Learn as much as you can about how you function, what your strengths and weaknesses are, and what you need to work better and smarter.

Then communicate those needs to the people you work with—not in a demanding manner, but with mutual respect and consideration. Ask, for example, "Would you be willing to make a trade with me? I am having real trouble getting myself organized to begin our project. I'd appreciate your making an outline for me to follow. Then I believe I can give you what you need."

Give those around you permission to get you back on track. Let others know it's OK to set limits on you, such as, "I really love hearing your stories, but we need to finish this job by 3:30. Please, no more stories for now." Your job is to say, "Thank you," when the limit is set. And for heaven's sake, don't take offense. Be grateful the other person cares enough about your work production that he is willing to set that limit. It means he respects what you have to contribute. Appreciate that respect.

Be clear with others if you simply cannot do some aspect of your job. It takes real courage to admit limitations, but know that you have so many positive skills and attributes that you have room to be less than perfect. We all are.

Even if you are hard to work with, admit it. "I know I'm a perfectionist. I suppose I'm hardest on myself, but I just want to get the best job done that's possible to do." Often when you are honest with others, you will find they will try their hardest to support you. At least you will be accepted as you are. The problem comes when you don't admit your limitations, and others get really sick of having to deal with them.

Finally, don't commit to anything you cannot or may not be able to do. If your time management is not under control, don't volunteer to drive to the airport. Instead, say, "I'd rather you drive. I don't want to take any chances that we miss the plane."

In the long run, you'll be respected for your honest assessment of yourself and your abilities. By taking responsibility and setting limits on yourself, you will reduce the stress you create for others and won't leave anyone in the lurch. Then, work away at building one skill at a time to overcome the effects of your ADD. Know that you are an asset rather than a stress producer.

8

Considering Career Changes

C hances are that every now and then you stop thinking about the day-to-day "busy-ness" of the workplace and ask yourself some larger questions: What do I really want to do with my life? What kind of work do I really want to do? How can I use my talents and gifts more fully? Most of the time, you're so busy with the daily grind of making a living that you may forget to dream and wonder. When on-the-job stress crushes down upon you, though, your dreams pop back up—a blessed escape from feeling that you've lost all hope of being happy—or you may try to find new ways to reduce that stress by expressing yourself outside of your work.

You begin to think that maybe you'll quit your job and open a fruit stand on the beach. You might decide that there is no way you can ever make a living doing what you really want to do, and you suddenly feel very, very old. Perhaps you find yourself wondering whether you might be able to go back to school and completely change your career path. Let's look at the real you and what your career options can be.

Developing Your Identity

At about age eighteen months, you started to become aware of who you were. You experienced an innate drive to discover your identity, a core component of human nature. That's why you appeared to be an insatiably possessive toddler who constantly yelled, "me," "mine," and "no." If only the adults around had known that this was your first voyage in your discovery of yourself, they wouldn't have worried that you would never learn to share!

For about the next eighteen months, you were naturally drawn to find out about yourself. You wanted to differentiate your nose from your daddy's nose. You wanted to show off how you could climb up on a chair and jump off. *You* could do that. You began to realize you had feelings, and those feelings changed from happy, to sad, to silly, to mad. By age three, you had a beginning data base that stored the components of your identity.

Though you continued to refine your identity throughout childhood, your attention was spread thin because of the many other things you were learning. When adolescence struck, the major focus of your attention shifted back to redefining your identity—this time, it was your identity in relation to the world outside your family and in comparison to your peers. Who am I? became a question that you asked yourself over and over again, probably well into your twenties. If you were lucky, you had found a large part of the answer by the time you reached adulthood and were on your way to living out your life.

However, if in early childhood or adolescence too much emphasis was placed on being a *good* little girl or boy, you may have only learned to automatically behave in the *right* way, which in many instances denied you the opportunity to develop who you really were and who you were to become.

How do you know who the true you is, or whether you are who you think you are naturally? Ask yourself whether you feel guilty for some of the things you want to do but don't because you "shouldn't" want them. Do you try to do what is sensible even though you are drawn to other interests? Does your choice of work feel as if it fits you?

All of these questions will give you a guide to determine whether you are your own person or more of a package of acceptable behaviors that you developed to get the approval of people around you.

Listen to the voice inside you that says, "I would really like to do ____, but I'd better not. What would people think?" Maybe the voice chastises you: "Shame on you for wanting to play all the time. You have to work first and play later." Perhaps the voice uses scare tactics like, "You'll never get anywhere in life if you don't settle down and quit _____." That inner voice is only a recording of things that were either said to you directly or taught to you as values.

Judith loves the job she has as a legal aide. She tells her best friend, Renee, "You should become a paralegal. It's a great job."

When Renee grimaces and says, "I'd have to do too much paper-work. I'd rather be a flight attendant," Judith argues with her, telling Renee all the reasons why she's wrong in her choice. What Judith fails to realize is that Renee isn't made like her, doesn't have the same interests or skills, and in fact would hate being a legal assistant. Though Judith means well, her advice is at best useless, and at worst bad, for Renee.

One young man I know decided he wanted to go into law enforce-ment. However, he knows himself well and immediately said, "I don't want to be a detective—too much paperwork, and I don't want to be inside a prison all day. I'd like to be a marshal, sheriff's deputy, or policeman who can be outside most of the time." This is a very good choice for him. It fits.

Every one of us has interests and skills that are inherent. We don't learn them, and we don't outgrow them—we were born with them. Sometimes we have skills without the interest to back them up. There seems to be a societal belief that we must use all the skills with which we've been blessed. I can tell you, though: if you don't have an interest in something, you'll be miserable doing it, whether you're skilled or not.

I am going to ask you to learn to listen to yourself and your desires. Ironically, I know you will be able to become more responsible if you do, rather than less.

Whether you are ADD or not, you probably have had many experi-ences that highlighted the discrepancy between what you like and want to do and what others think you should do. Words like "be responsible" and "be sensible" are often used to try to convince you to do something someone else wants. When you factor being ADD into the equation, there is even a bigger schism between who you naturally are and what has been expected of you. Since you had little opportunity during your school years to be accepted as you are naturally made, you may have spent a great deal of time feeling like a misfit. Well, you are not. You just don't fit someone else's idea of how people should be.

One of the most wonderful aspects of working with ADD over the last ten years has been the discovery that there is a fabulous segment of our population that was hidden away trying to make it in disguise—and that includes me. Now we can surface in all our glory, with our strengths as well as our difficulties in hand, to make our contributions to the world.

In the process of taking hold of our true identities, we often need to change the way we think about ourselves. Just because you didn't fit comfortably into your work environment until now, doesn't mean you can't fit. Nor does it mean you are a *mis*fit.

For example, when Rita failed to do well in clerical work, she almost gave up working. She was able to rely on her husband's income for support. And besides, what could she do?

It wasn't until she became bored hanging around the house watching TV that she discovered the true Rita. Besides watching TV, Rita liked to talk on the phone—a lot. A friend of hers heard of a women's shelter that needed winter clothing the residents could wear on job interviews. Rita got on the phone. In one morning, she made all the arrangements to collect wearable clothing in good condition in a variety of sizes. That same afternoon, she picked the clothing up, drove it over to the shelter, and was back home before dinner.

That evening, her husband instantly noticed a change in Rita's mood. "Hey, what's up?" he asked. "You're happier than I've seen you in ages."

Rita was surprised, but when she thought about his comment, she realized he was right. She was happy—very happy.

The next day, as she sat down to watch her soap operas, she felt an enormous urge to turn the TV off and replicate the good feelings from the day before. TV suddenly seemed very boring to her. Just then the phone rang: it was the shelter. They wanted to thank her. One woman had already found a job; four others were out looking. All were admiring their new clothes, the first they'd had in a long time. The director wanted Rita to know what a big help she'd been.

"Is there anything else I can do to help you?" Rita asked. The director, delighted, invited her to a volunteer orientation.

Four years later, with a degree in social work under her belt, Rita now works in a women's program for abuse recovery, teaches job skills classes, and directs several charitable drives each year. She is happy, vibrant, and successful.

Rita remembers that when she was a little girl, she wanted to help people. Whenever she said that aloud, however, she had been told she'd better learn to help herself first. After all, her grades were poor, she couldn't pay attention in class, and no one thought she would be able to make much of a contribution to the world, especially one that required further schooling. But they were wrong: Rita just had to find her fit.

Sometimes we hear advice in our minds that doesn't feel right, advice about how we should act or the kind of work we should do, but we don't always trust our own negative feelings about it.

For example, from the time Melvin was very young, his dad taught him that he needed to prepare for a job as an officer in the armed forces. That's what Melvin's father had done, and his grandfather, and his great-grandfather. Melvin tried very hard to convince himself that he wanted to do this. He would talk to himself, saying, "General, plan this campaign; round up your troops; sign this paper."

All the while, Melvin had a secret dream. He loved the theater, and when he wasn't trying to be a general, he was designing stage scenery, putting plays on in his mind, and directing his friends in neighborhood productions. In high school he spent every free hour working in the school theater, so much so that his father threatened to send him to military school if he didn't spend more time on his studies.

Melvin felt terribly guilty about what he was doing. He thought there was something wrong with him because he loved theater so much. He thought he shouldn't feel the way he did. So, Melvin quit working in theater and buried himself in his preparation for a "sensible career"—the one his father had chosen for him. Over the years, whenever something reminded him of his childhood dreams, he felt guilty. Secretly, he was never able to get past the worry that something was wrong with him.

Though Melvin had an adequate career in the service, he did not shine and definitely did not become a general. Only after he retired did he allow himself to indulge in some volunteer work at the community theater. There he found that he actually had talent and support from others who shared his interest. The voice in his mind finally quieted, and Melvin felt like he was at home at last.

When we consider the elements that go into developing our identities, we can really take some commonsense lessons from gardening. If a plant needs an acidic soil in order to flourish, no one is surprised when it withers if planted in alkaline soil. You can doctor it endlessly in the alkaline soil, but it will still end up in a weakened condition. You know this, and you wouldn't try to force that plant beyond its limits.

Can you say the same for yourself?

Developing Your ADD Identity

Your first reaction to discovering you have ADD was probably something like "Oh, that's why I am the way I am!" Accompanied by that sense of relief, you began to get used to a new identity.

Until you were diagnosed with ADD, you probably suffered from feeling different without knowing that there was a tangible reason for that difference, a difference that was generally not thought to be OK. Once the ADD diagnosis was made, you could define yourself in a new way. The relief you felt with "Oh, that's what I've got" was the first stage in the development of your new identity.

Shortly after that sense of relief, you probably began to feel sadness. This second stage of identity development was a grief reaction because your discovery meant that you were leaving something behind on your way to your new identity. What you were leaving behind were the beliefs that shaped your life previously, your lost potential, and the hurts and traumas that came because you couldn't be what others thought you should be.

Go ahead and do your grieving. Grief is a normal, natural part of growth and change, necessary if you are to release the past to make way for the future. If you feel sad, cry. If you feel angry, talk about that anger and reconnect with the dreams that lie underneath it. If you feel depressed, open your heart and hopes so you can see what you're really made of. Finally, acknowledge that it is time to move forward to find the new you, having put the old, outdated, prediscovered inauthentic you to rest.

Stage three calls for you to find others like yourself. Together you will rejoice in your similarities, support one another, and teach each other in a language that you all understand.

I'm always reminded of the children's story of a lion that is raised in a flock of sheep. This lion can never quite learn how to say "baaa" just the right way. Although the lion is tolerated and even loved by the flock, the other sheep are aware of his differences and wonder about him. He spends all his time trying to roar softly.

Then one day he comes upon a pride of lions. He hears one of them roar and opens his eyes wide. It sounded like him, but much bigger. How wonderful! The lions greet him, take him in and give him permission to roar as loudly as he wishes. It takes a little time for him to get used to the new ways, but he takes to them readily once he feels it's okay. He becomes happy, and the sheep are happy for him, too. He has found his fit—just like we all need to do.

Stage four involves experimenting and experiencing in order to find out what the new, real you is made of. As if needing to try out a whole new set of skills, you need to discover what you can do, what you like, and how you are. Doing this experimenting with others like you will be a wonderful experience. You learn to cope with and control your ADD in some areas of your life, and you learn to let it loose in others.

Throughout this process, which usually takes about a year and a half, your job is to stay aware and be nonjudgmental. Be an observer and collect your observations to examine. You'll learn from your reactions to all sorts of things.

Finally, you are ready to summarize your findings and answer the important question, Who am I with my ADD under control? At this point you will need to look at your environment, and that includes your job. Does your job fit you? Does your style of living fit you? Are you in the right place for you?

It's an exciting time. It can be a little scary because you may find you need to change some things. Trust yourself and know that you can make any changes you wish, and you don't have to make any changes you don't want to make.

If you were diagnosed as a child *and* trained to understand and use your ADD to your advantage, you would already have gone through these five stages to knowing yourself as a person with ADD. You would be used to yourself and, hopefully, comfortable with yourself.

I mentioned earlier that a young man I know found out as a child that he was ADD. Mory's parents were forthright and clear about what ADD is and what it means. He was taught that it was one of the many ways in which people are wired, and the development of his natural skills received as much attention as the skills that were more difficult for him to achieve. He did not make phenomenal grades in school, but he did learn to study, a little at a time.

As an Outwardly Expressive ADD person, Mory was supported in the cultivation of friendships, had some experience in radio during his teen years, and learned to run the technical board. He was active in sports and was encouraged to spend time working at jobs that proved to him he was able to do many things. He saw a whole world outside of school that allowed him to learn that not everyone has to be a scholar to succeed.

By the time Mory graduated from high school, he knew the kinds of help he needed to accommodate his ADD. He knew what he needed to do so he wouldn't shoot himself in the foot, so to speak. He had basic study skills. Maybe most importantly, Mory liked who he was and felt hopeful about the future.

He wanted to get a college education because he felt it would be an advantage to him in the future, but he also knew he hated bookwork. With his parents' support, he decided to continue in sports while going to college. Mory described his decision to play sports this way: "It gives me something to look forward to while I'm having to do all kinds of things I don't like."

Not only did he continue in sports and eventually make the varsity team, but Mory is due to finish college in another semester with a decent grade point average. It took him an extra year, and it wasn't always easy for him, but he's finishing.

Because he knew himself well and was familiar with the ins and outs of his ADD, Mory had already learned how to stick with something he wanted to achieve. He knew what to put his effort into and when to withdraw from a direction that didn't suit him. Fortunately, he also found a major he's very excited about.

In considering life after school, Mory knew he wanted a job in which he had mobility, could use his physicality, could deal with people, and would not get bored doing the same thing day in and day out, because stimulation is important to him. Mory is emotionally and physically powerful, protective of people, very perceptive, compassionate, and he wanted to make a difference in the world. In law enforcement, Mory believes he's found a career that fits him.

When Mory realized this would be a great job for him, he became very excited, so excited that he suddenly pulled out all the stops and wanted to make great grades. He even considered studying on the weekend for the first time. To everyone's surprise, especially his own, he told his family, "Can you believe I've spent my whole life trying to get out of school, and now I'm thinking about going to graduate school?" Everyone had a good laugh, with a few tears in the corners of their eyes. How wonderful when someone finds something that fits him!

If You Were Diagnosed as an Adult

Because ADD has been seen in a moral light for so long before being found to be neurochemically based, many undiagnosed adults feel guilty because they were told, "You could do it if you just tried." People who feel such a tremendous amount of guilt don't live with joy, nor do they tend to seek out what fits them. Instead, they tend to hide what gives them joy if it doesn't fit the program they believe they must conform to, lying to themselves and everyone else about their true natures. Their self-esteem tends to be pretty poor.

Not valuing yourself, you are likely to deny yourself the option to do what you desire. Even if you were diagnosed with ADD as a child, you are likely to have grown up confused or on a track that is less than great for you, unless you were guided to know your value and strengths so you could use your ADD to advantage.

Blanche was diagnosed as ADD at age ten, placed on medication for two years, then taken off medication as she entered adolescence. Her life fell apart as school became more demanding, and she became less attentive. Her poor grades kept her out of extracurricular activities, and she felt very poor about herself.

She tried to go to college but couldn't concentrate on anything for very long. Blanche changed her major three times in eighteen months and finally dropped out of school before she finished her sophomore year. She tried secretarial school, went to beauty school, and finally took a job as a messenger. At age twenty-four, she is still lost, doesn't know how to get out of the trap she finds herself in, and has no idea what she is good at or even what she likes.

At this point Blanche not only needs to be reevaluated for ADD, she needs to be trained in relation to being ADD. Then she will need some help in figuring out who she is, what she likes, and where her talents lie. She'll need training to assist her in developing good habits that she missed out on over the years—study habits and living skills, such as how to keep her apartment straight and her bank account under control.

Finally, Blanche needs counseling to improve her self-esteem. Only then will she be able to live up to the potential that is within her—the potential that has been overlooked because no one knew how to help her, including herself.

Then there's Morris, age sixty-three, who shot out of the counseling room, thrust his arm upward in a salute, and yelled, "Yes!" Morris had just found out that he is ADD. "No wonder life has been so hard," he said. "I'm gonna find out who I am and do what I want to do."

Morris is retired and is determined to make up for lost time. Though outwardly successful, he feels that all he has done in his life is work, just to keep up. With tears starting to well up in his eyes, Morris said, "You know, I always wanted to do so many exciting things, but I never had time. I couldn't take the time, or I'd get behind. I thought I was just a little slower than most, but now I realize I have a lot to learn about myself. Maybe there are some things I'm not so slow at.

"I want to hike, climb, and spend lots of time outdoors. Then I want to help other people get to do these things a lot earlier than I did. Maybe I'll teach a continuing education class or start a program for wilderness exploration. Or, maybe, I'll be able to find a partner to get a retreat going. I can do the outdoor stuff, and a partner could handle the paperwork and business end. At any rate, I have a new lease on life—thanks to finding out I'm ADD."

How to Find Your Fit

Throughout this chapter I've stressed how important it is to find your fit, how to make the choices and find the lifestyle that's right for you. That's how you come to feel good about yourself and what you're doing with your life. No one can be truly happy doing something that doesn't fit, and the repercussions create ill feelings and ill health.

You need to fit into your work life as much as you do your personal life. After all, you not only spend a lot of hours every day on the job, but a lot of your sense of accomplishment and feelings of success come from the work you do. So, you need to be sure that you set things up to achieve what you want.

A simple rule for finding your fit involves doing what you like to do and avoiding what you don't.

Yet, even as I write these words, I can hear the uproar: "You can't always do what you want to do. Life won't let you."

I counter those all-too-familiar statements by replying, "If you believe life should be hard, you will make it hard for yourself. If you believe it is OK for you to do what you like or love to do, as long as you remain a responsible and contributing member of society, you will tend to find opportunities to do what you like." In my opinion, too much time is wasted trying to do what doesn't fit, but you'll have to make up your own mind about that.

There is one major difficulty in following the philosophy of doing what you like and avoiding what you don't: you have to face the grief you feel over all the time you spent doing what others said you should do, or what you believed you had to do. That can be a lot of time lost. The sooner you come to grips with your past, though, let go of it, and do what fits, the sooner you'll be happy. As a lawyer friend once said to me, "Take your lumps and go on with your life." That's great advice.

I know one woman named Sarah who was taught that women shouldn't drive trucks. Yet she loved the open road, being on the go, and seeing the countryside. What she most wanted to do was drive an eighteen-wheeler, but she never talked to anyone about her desire because she was afraid they would laugh at her. Instead she took a desk job processing invoices for a wholesaler.

One day, almost five years after she took the job, a call came in saying that one of the drivers would be dropping off a corrected invoice sheet that needed immediate attention. When the driver arrived, Sarah was shocked: the driver was a woman. Sarah was so surprised that she began to argue with the woman. "Women can't be drivers," she said.

"I've been driving for five years," the woman answered. "I started right after the company began hiring women. I always wanted to be a driver, so I just took the training and applied for the job. They hired me, and I love it."

Sarah's inner desire was right for her, but she had suppressed it because she had been told she shouldn't pay attention to it. *Wrong.* Worse yet, she felt so afraid that people would call her stupid for having missed a chance, that she never did let anyone know about her dream. Nor did she do anything to become a truck driver. Instead, Sarah kept processing invoices—and taking medication for depression.

Now, does that make any sense to you? Wouldn't it have made more sense for Sarah to have followed her heart and applied for the job she'd always wanted? Sarah had decided that she would not be allowed to do what she really wanted to do, and that's exactly the path she followed.

You don't have to make your choices like that. You can decide to follow your dream and find a job that fits you.

Avoid people who repeatedly put down your ideas. They don't know how much harm they are doing. They are probably trying to protect you in some way, but stay away from them if they can't see what brings you happiness.

Instead, spend your time around people who are supportive of you, people who enjoy the same things that you do. Try many, many, many things. Experience different jobs in different settings. Then analyze what you like and what you don't like about the jobs. You will soon find a pattern.

Anytime you get an urge to do something, there is a reason. You may not understand how the desire connects to your search for your fit, but I promise you, there are no mistakes. There's something in the experience that you need to know. You will learn, discovering some piece of your special pattern. At the same time you pursue the urge, think about what you are doing, analyze the fit for you, and consider how the particular experience applies to your study of yourself.

I am not saying that you should haphazardly follow every whim, a tendency for some people with ADD. I am saying that you should thoughtfully pursue interests that catch your attention.

A.K. was a home builder who loved to construct rustic homes. When one of his customers shared an interest in doing wood sculpture, A.K. mentioned that he'd always thought he'd like to try his hand at some chain-saw sculpting but figured people would think he was foolish.

His customer urged him to go to a woodworking club, and he did.

To his surprise, A.K. found a lot of people there like himself, people who loved wood. He discovered an outlet for creativity he didn't even know he had until then, yet he had almost discounted his desire because he thought it was foolish.

Even if you don't yet know what your desire or dream is, you can start finding it by asking questions. Talk to people about their jobs and ask them how they got where they are. Find out what attracted them to the businesses they're in. See if you hear anything that excites you, that seems to fit you. Then be sure to ask each person you talk with for five more names of people with whom you can talk. Networking is very important when you are trying to discover your fit.

As part of the process of discovering your fit, try constructing a time line to jog your memory. On a piece of paper, draw a horizontal line. On the left end put a dot and label it "birth." On the far right put another dot labeled with your current age. Then divide the intervening space into four- or five-year segments.

Next, mark the times when you were really, really happy and write in what job, hobby, or interest you were pursuing at that point. Don't discount anything as being unimportant or off the track. If it comes to mind, it belongs in this exercise. Now look at the common thread that runs through your happy times.

When Jenna did her time line, she discovered two things that had brought her great joy: dancing as a child and creating a program for teenagers to build self-esteem.

Though she'd worked as a very successful executive director for years, Jenna was beginning to prepare for a change in her life. Doing her time line allowed her to see the importance of being creative and artistically expressive. She began to consider shifting her emphasis to creative projects that included writing and program development, perhaps training that incorporated movement. Not yet complete with her transition, Jenna is on her way to finding her fit for the next chapter of her life.

Recognizing and Dealing with the "Shoulds"

Many people with ADD are in the wrong profession or job because the ADD style of wiring predisposes them to be good at creative tasks, and our culture has a belief that people can't make a living in creative fields. Someone forgot to tell Walt Disney and George Lucas, however.

Also, when the word *creative* is used in conjunction with career choices, an image of a painter or a craftsman comes to most people's minds. However, creativity is a way of approaching any work. It is putting things together in a fresh way, whether those things are materials, ideas, programs, or anything else. Creativity does not pertain to just arts and crafts.

Some of the things that people with ADD do best—the creative, entrepreneurial types of things—are generally considered risky. "Yes, I'm glad you like to take photographs, but you can't make a living that way. What you *should* do is . . ." Or, "You want to be a painter? That's nice—what a great hobby—but you have to get a real job. Here's what you *should* do . . . " How many times have we heard these things? Even if no one is saying those exact words to you, they are in the air or floating around in your mind.

I am here to tell you that you can make a good living using your creative interests and talents, no matter what they are, *if* you are willing to become good at your craft, to network, and to work hard. It may take you longer than you'd like to build your business or find the right slot in the workplace, or it may not, but if you don't give up, you'll find your niche.

If you would like to change how your thinking and behavior are shaped and give yourself the freedom to follow your dreams, you can. Just face the "shoulds" head on. Use your good brain to decide whether you still want to do what you were once taught you *should* do. Would you rather make a change and do something you were taught you *shouldn't* do?

You, and no one else, are in charge of your life.

Sarah didn't realize this. When she found out that women could work as truck drivers and that her own employer hired them, she could have asked herself whether or not she would still like to be one. Then her job would have been to listen carefully to whatever she was feeling inside. If she felt guilty, then she would know a "should" was operating. If she felt a twinge of pleasure at the thought, she would know that she still held a desire to drive. If she felt afraid, she would need to realize that fear keeps her from knowing what she would like to do. That fear is trying to tell her something, even though she might not know exactly what it was. Fear does not necessarily mean she doesn't want to drive; it might only mean that she's afraid of disapproval.

To overcome the fear, Sarah would have needed to ask herself, What is the worst thing that could happen if I gave driving a try? She might have found that what she most feared was being made fun of for having such a "silly" idea. Then she could have decided if she was willing to risk the worst possible scenario. Once she made a purposeful decision either way—whether to try driving or to stick with her desk job—she would have been in charge of her life, and her depression would have disappeared.

If she decided to give driving a try, Sarah would not need to instantly quit her job. Instead, she could take a number of steps to determine how she really felt about truck driving. Never really having done it, she could begin to talk to people who were in the business, asking what they liked and disliked about it. She could interview people who hired truck drivers to find out what kind of jobs are available and what her prospective bosses would be like.

If Sarah liked what she heard, she could inquire about driving schools and find out whether she could use her vacation time or evenings or weekends to acquire the skills she needed. Once trained, she could go on a trip with someone before quitting her job totally. That way she'd find out what life was like on the road. Finally, Sarah could resign her job after locating another one in her new field.

Never forget that all decisions are changeable. If after six months or a year, Sarah didn't like driving as much as she thought she would, she could always go back to office work. Granted, she might not be able to work for the same company, but she would be able to find a job. If she did go back to office work, it would be with a satisfied heart, knowing she had followed her dream and made a positive decision to come back to work she preferred.

ADD and Career Options: What Works Well

Certain kinds of jobs work well for people who are ADD. That doesn't mean you can't take another kind of job. Nor does it mean you are locked into doing only a few kinds of things. Typically, however, more people with ADD go into certain fields or subspecialty areas than others.

What you are trying to do is match your strengths and the demands and requirements of the job. Remember that the most important thing for you to know is how you feel in your heart about a job or a particular type of work. If you have a strong desire in your heart, you can make just about anything happen. If you want something badly enough, then that is probably what fits for you—even if it isn't a typical match for someone with your style of ADD.

Let's look at career and job options that typically fit each type of ADD.

People with Outwardly Expressive ADD need opportunities to be expressive, mobile, and outwardly directed. Sales fits the criteria perfectly. Sales jobs come in many forms, from retail sales to selling yourself as a personality. In this line of work, you can be a part of a sales team, work by yourself, or direct sales training. You might be selling the latest research project to a university dean or selling times shares for a condominium, but your charisma, gift of gab, sense of humor, ability to read people like a book, and all-around great people skills will tend to make you successful.

Many Outwardly Expressive ADD people start their own businesses. These entrepreneurs often arrive at the cutting edge of innovation at just the right time, starting trends and making way for something new. If you are this type of person, your enormous energy is used well in taking risks that others wouldn't even consider. Yet, you don't see them as such tremendous risks, for you believe so strongly and work so hard that you make things work out.

It didn't take me long to discover that many of the people who interview me about ADD are, in fact, ADD themselves. The media, especially radio and television, are filled with people who have Outwardly Expressive ADD. Entertainers and other performers almost always have a lot of this type of wiring, especially the more flamboyant ones. Highly successful teachers and speakers often benefit from this tendency, too.

Many careers allow you to bring these talents to the table. For example, you can be a lawyer who uses dramatics in the courtroom, or a law enforcement officer who uses his or her expressiveness to advantage. Perhaps you'd like to be social worker or counselor but don't want to sit in an office all the time. In that case, you might find work in a residential rural setting or use the techniques of psychodrama and art therapy. Perhaps you would introduce these methods in a business setting where they had never been used before.

If you are somewhat hyperactive, that must also be factored into your career choices. If you're considering a career as a driver, for example, you might be better off driving race cars and motorcycles than sitting at the wheel of a big rig, hauling cargo long distances. Selling products person to person, so that you could move around quite a bit, would be a much better fit for you than doing phone sales.

If you are Outwardly Expressive ADD, your style of operating can fit into many settings. All you have to do is know yourself, then find the place to use your talents. Wherever you're working now, consider other ways you can showcase who you are and what you like to do. If you think about it, you'll find many opportunities.

When things go right for you folks with Outwardly Expressive

ADD, they go *very* right. You often emerge as a leader in your profession or trade. You have found your fit, and everyone knows it.

People with Inwardly Directed ADD tend to use their talents and abilities in more quiet and subtle ways than their Outwardly Expressive counterparts. Preferring to work alone or behind the scenes, they focus attention on what they are doing rather than on who they are.

Inwardly Directed ADD people are likely to utilize creativity with a focus on a specific talent. You may find yourself drawn to arts and crafts, photography, video, film, multimedia projects, and all types of design work. You'd probably be very happy in one of these fields and do quite well. Truly, you can make a living doing what you love.

As you quietly nurture your skills and talents, you will want to be with people who are similar to you, and that will prove to be good for networking. Jobs transfer from one medium to another. Whole groups of creative people work in tandem, referring business to others with slightly different skills.

I'm reminded of a photographer friend of mine who sometimes serves as the creative director for projects. He is likely to need video or film skills, computer graphics, a storyboard layout for a book, or creative writing for a project. The person who has the film capability may come upon a project that needs still photography, and she refers my friend for the job. Meanwhile, the computer graphics person recommends both of them to the company he is doing advertising layout for, because the company has another project requiring their skills. And so it goes.

The business is there. It's only that many people unfamiliar with advertising, publishing, and creative work don't realize it. Find out if this is your interest.

When you find your fit, you are likely to be a part of a creative team, formally or informally, that produces some very nice work. You can become quite well known for your talents, though attention is not what you particularly want. Time and opportunity to create is all that matters to you. You would be like a caged animal doing anything else, your spirit suppressed.

Inwardly Directed ADD people also tend to gravitate toward technical and mechanical skills, from the inventors and mechanics of the world to the modern-day techies who love nothing better than a problem to solve. These folks love to talk shop with others who know what they are talking about, whether it's repairing cars, building machine parts, or developing software.

When things go right for you and you find your fit, you quietly enjoy life. Happy to be able to spend time doing what you are doing, you may be less interested in creating a business empire or making lots of money than in being able to do what you love. That's not to say you don't know how to spend money, but you may put the money you make into your work, buying more equipment or enlarging your workspace.

If you are not working in your area of interest, the likelihood of your becoming depressed is extremely high, and anxiety would haunt you. You need to express yourself through your work in your own way in order to live life fully.

Another category of work that many people with Inwardly Expressive ADD pursue and excel in involves some form of "people work." Teachers, social workers, counselors, and people who work with children and animals fall into this category. The core trait that contributes to an interest in this field is hypersensitivity, which yields compassion, caring, and good listening skills.

If you are drawn in this direction, you probably spent a lot of time being a good friend to others even before you chose a profession. Able to empathize with others' situations, your quietness allows you to listen well, rather than taking over the situation and trying to fix it, though you certainly don't mind helping to fix things.

When plying your trade, you tend to form long-lasting relationships. Loyalty to your charges is foremost in your mind. Often highly dedicated, you may put others before yourself. You truly care what happens to the other guy, and your reward is that person's success.

When you can't work at what you love, often because your ADD has gotten in the way of your getting the degrees needed to do the job you want to do, you tend to bring your interest into whatever job you have. You may also turn ordinary relationships into therapeutic encounters. Many modern-day support groups have people who fall into this category. Volunteerism is also a way in which you can do what you do well without formal education. I find it unfortunate that the training required for much of this helping kind of work is not more experientially based. This would allow a person to work professionally in a field he loves.

The biggest hindrance your ADD brings to this kind of work is difficulty knowing when to stop, getting overinvolved with a client or customer, and ultimately burning out. You must have a life on the side that meets personal needs, so that you don't have to get everything out of your work. But then, you probably love your work so much that you often don't want to stop.

Outdoor careers are also attractive to people with Inwardly Directed ADD. From the forestry service, to farming, geology, to being a game warden, working outdoors can be so important to some people that they cringe at the thought of having to spend much time inside. Though these careers are not always easy to come by, they are worth pursuing if you are drawn to them. You may also want to consider self-employment in some type of landscape work. From tree trimming to gardening, stone laying, installing water fountains, or tending golf greens, the inveterate outdoorsman must have freedom.

One woman I know with Inwardly Directed ADD, a mother of four, lived in a large city but desperately wanted to work outside. She solved her situation by establishing a business in which she took care of indoor plants in office buildings. Though the job wasn't perfect—she did have to go inside—she was still able to be among plants, which reminded her of the out-of-doors, and she enjoyed traveling from building to building. The hours even fit her schedule as a mom.

It's not surprising that people with Highly Structured ADD are drawn to careers with innate structure, such as in accounting, the sciences, financial planning, or the military. Flowcharts, computer programs, and scientific research protocols all are grist for the Highly Structured mill. Keeping track of a million details, if a network for structuring those details is already in place, makes people with Highly Structured ADD comfortable.

If you have Highly Structured ADD, you must believe in what you are doing—but once you do, you will tend not to vary one bit. In the right job, such as the comptroller of a large company, you are a godsend, and your employer will recognize that. You often provide the glue that holds everything else together.

Many people with ADD are a blend of two or more types, and many jobs have more than one aspect to them. The trick is to put the person together with the type of job that honors the balance of talents.

Consider a man named Joe and his job as a home builder. Joe is an artisan with a creative eye. He builds homes that he literally fashions on the spot with nothing but the simplest of working plans to guide him. He can be found with his head cocked back, considering some way to make the angle of the house's roof pitch just right so that it both looks good architecturally and holds up well under the stress of bad weather and years of wear and tear. An ADD person who is mostly Inwardly Directed with both artistic and mechanical ability, Joe is also partly Highly Structured ADD. The combination works well for him.

Many highly trained professionals are a combination of Outwardly Expressive and Inwardly Directed ADD along with a goodly amount of Highly Structured ADD. The latter seems necessary to survive the large amounts of school necessary for many professions; the other components shape the subspecialty pursued. For example, a physician who goes into public health work might be Inwardly Directed and Highly Structured. In contrast, an emergency room physician would probably be Outwardly Expressive and Highly Structured. Any combination is possible.

Most jobs and careers have room for more than one type of ADD to exist. There are as many types of doctors as there are types of medical care. Precision surgery requires different talents and skills from family practice. Lawyers, too, vary from flamboyant trial attorneys to empathetic family law practitioners to precise tax attorneys. Every profession has considerable variance, so you no doubt can find a subspecialty that you like and in which you can excel.

Should You Change Jobs?

Maybe, maybe not.

This is a difficult question to answer—for anyone. There are always some unknowns. To help you in this decision, answer this question first: Would you like to stay in the kind of work you're in if you could fix some of the problems you are having?

If you answer yes, then you know you are basically satisfied with your work choice, and you can draw from the various chapters in this book for help with specific issues. If you like what you do but don't think you can, or don't want to, fix certain aspects of your present situation, you might want to consider changing companies, trying self-employment, or taking your skills and applying them to a different but related line of work.

If, however, you feel you've been trapped in a prison for years, disliking or even hating what you do; feel sad; or feel depressed about not using a talent, gift, or interest, then I'd strongly recommend changing what you do to make a living. To a large degree your choice will depend upon how strongly you feel about what you are doing. Add in how bad you feel about what you are doing, and you will have created some guidelines.

If you are staying in a job because you're afraid you can't make it anywhere else, then you're staying for the wrong reason. You need to begin the process of leaving that job, with some counseling, if necessary.

Timing is another factor to consider. If you have just bought a new house, have a new baby, and recently finished school, you may want to stay with what you are doing for a while. However, if your kids are grown, your debts are limited, and your spouse is agreeable, why not change?

Most people feel they fall somewhere between these two scenarios. Regardless of your life circumstances, you can measure how you feel inside. It's your feelings that will make your emotional and physical health good or bad, not your mind, logic, or what someone else tells you to do. To help you measure your feelings, read the following statements and check the one ones that pertain to you:

1. _____ I like what I do in general, but I don't like certain specific things about my job.

2. _____ I will work at fixing what is wrong with my job. (If you mark this one, decide how long you are willing to try fixing it: I will set a time limit of _____. At the end of this time, begin a transition process.)

3. _____ I don't want to try any longer. (If you mark this one, begin the transition right away.)

4. _____ This is not a good time for me to make a job move. (If you mark this one, figure out what would make it a better time and write that down: _____

5. _____ My outside time limit for making a change is _____

6. _____ On a scale of 1 to 10, I feel miserable (1) or wonderful (10) about my job.
(The lower the score, the more urgent it is that you change. If you score 5 to 8, you need to shift what you are doing or the way in which you are doing your job, but the urgency isn't there. If you score 8 or 9, you just need to make some minor adjustments. If you score 10, say "thank you," and don't change a thing.)

You deserve to work in the way that fits you at something that you love. Anything less is worth your time and energy to fix so you can be all you can be.

Sometimes it takes a while to move the pieces of your life around, but I believe in you, and I know you can do it.

9

Self-Employment and ADD

E thel remembers selling lemonade from a booth on her front lawn when she was six years old. By twelve, she had established herself in a baby-sitting business with four regular weekly customers. At thirteen, she set her sights on winning a prize for the most wrapping paper sold in a citywide drive to raise money so that low-income children could go to summer camp.

Now, at 36, Ethel continues walking the path of self-employment. To be sure, she tried working for a company after college, but it lasted only a year and a half. The urge to be her own boss never went away. Even though she was in charge of opening a new branch for her company, she constantly thought about projects and businesses of her own that she wanted to try.

Ethel is the epitome of the self-employed entrepreneur. She loves the freedom. She has plenty of ideas of her own to pursue and never gets bored. And she doesn't worry about someone having power over her; no one can ever fire her.

Are Ethel's feelings foreign to you? Do you like to receive a salary while someone else worries about the details and the ups and downs of the business? Or do you feel just like Ethel? Have you felt this way as long as you can remember? In your heart, have you always wanted to own your own business?

Though it's not for everyone, owning your own business might be just the thing for you, as it is for many people with ADD. Let's take a look at the reality of being your own boss, first the positives, then the negatives.

Self-Employment: The Reality

Freedom to choose your own direction is the greatest positive aspect of being self-employed. You can choose whether to have a physical place of business, provide a service, or manufacture a product. You can choose to open a shop you go to daily or to work out of your home. You can choose to work alone or to employ others. You have lots of options.

With a home-based business, you may be able to live anywhere because of the technological advances available today. Often all you need is a phone, fax, computer, modem, E-mail, or whatever else is invented tomorrow.

The rush, or high, of being in charge creates a wonderful power trip, in a positive way. You're it, the top dog. That doesn't mean you are a power maniac; it just means that the power and control you have feels good. Of course, along with power comes lots of responsibility.

Whatever dreams your mind imagines, you can implement. You can, within reason, be a "creativity junkie," trying this or that. You can come up with ten new designs or forty new ideas in one day, let them roll around in your head, sleep on them overnight, then have the privilege of deciding which of them you want to pursue. If you don't like any of them the next day, you can dream more. If you've already chosen a couple of new projects and something better comes along, you can change your priorities and do the new one that you like more.

Then there's the rush of cutting your own deals. Nothing else like it exists in the whole world, according to many self-employed entrepreneurs. You've dreamed something new, figured out what needs to be done, brought people together to implement it, and watched the completion of something that only a short while ago didn't exist. You've used your influence to share your dream with others, and they decide to buy in on it. Yes!

No one tells you what to do when you're in business for yourself. What a sense of power! You don't have to spend a lot of energy fitting into someone else's patterns, ways of doing things, and expectations. You don't have to be evaluated by someone who has authority over you.

Finally, you can pick and choose the people you want to do business with, both in terms of customers and coworkers. If you don't get along with someone, you don't have to work with them. You can find the optimal partners and companions to reflect who you are and what you want.

As any entrepreneur can tell you, however, being in business for yourself is not all fun and games. Yes, it's true that you're top dog and no one tells you what to do, but there are times when that is exactly the problem. Alone, you have no one to turn to who "truly knows what to do." Even if you have a partner, you have to judge for yourself what you feel is the right thing to do. You may find out quite quickly that no sure answers exist for some problems. Also, when things go wrong, guess who gets to take the responsibility.

Sure, you can hire outside consultation, but ultimately, if you're the boss, the buck stops with you. Other people cannot tell you what to do: they can only advise you. If things go wrong, it will be you who takes the blow on the jaw, not the consultant who gave you his best professional opinion.

For many people who are self-employed, isolation creates a problem. If the type of work you are doing is a one-person operation, you're on the road a lot, or you work at a creative or mental task, you might find that you spend many hours and days by yourself. Without coworkers to bounce ideas off of, complain to, or rejoice with, you could become lonely. You might want to consider setting up a support network with people in similar businesses or professions or with other people who are self-employed to alleviate some of that aloneness.

The fact that no one will be standing over you and telling you what to do is great. On the other hand, if no one forces you to get your work done, will you? You must be self-motivated and very disciplined if you are to be a success. Once the excitement of putting the deal together wears off, you may discover that settling down to do the very task you just created is much less fun. That's because the deal-cutting phase is creative, while the implementation of the dream is administrative. These are very different tasks, and often the same person doesn't do both well. Still, you must get the total job done if you are to stay in business.

I know about this particular problem only too well. Several years ago, I had the idea for a product, the one and only one I've ever developed. Being a committed self-employed entrepreneur most of my adult life, I rejoiced at the task of developing the product. After a year of creative work, mock-ups, and trial-and-error testing, the first batch of fifty rolled off my home assembly line. The very minute the last one was finished, I realized that I wanted to be in neither the manufacturing, marketing, nor distribution business. I had been thriving on the creativity of development and design; once that phase was completed, I was no longer interested. Ouch!

Another aspect of being self-employed is that you get to do *all* the jobs yourself, at least until you're able to hire people to do them for you. I'm not just talking about advertising and bookkeeping—I mean sweeping the floor and cleaning the bathrooms. No matter what the business is, whether it's service- or product-related, you get to do it all.

I'm reminded of the look of horror on the face of the manicurist who held her chipped nails out for me to see. Though hers were normally as beautifully groomed as those of her customers, she had just finished scrubbing spilled food off the carpet in the waiting room of her shop. Chocolate ground in the carpet by a child who had accompanied one of her customers, ketchup and mustard from a teenage client's burger, and spilled coffee from several of her customers had led her to a frenzy of cleaning. She moaned something about "having to do it all," while apologizing for the look of her hands. Clearly, she thought she had gone into business to do nails—not carpets.

Grant, a trained mental health professional, loved to do counseling. As soon as he gained enough experience, he decided to go into business for himself. He knew he had enough expertise about the different mental health conditions and treatments to stand on his own two feet. What he forgot about was that he had to get the clients to come in the door. Having always worked in clinics with established clientele, he'd only had to walk in and counsel.

Grant discovered he had to keep detailed financial records, book appointments, decide when to have people pay and when to wait for insurance payments, do his own clerical work, order magazine subscriptions, find office space with evening access, decorate the office, choose the music—and so on and so on. On top of that, he had to keep up with his continuing education and stay on top of new treatment forms and trends. Finally, he had to spend time counseling.

If you are in business for yourself, not only do you have to do all the jobs, you have to do them day after day after day. You don't get promoted; you are right where you're going to be: the boss.

In many businesses, activity and income are predictably cyclical; in some months income is high, in others it's low. However, the bills continue, regardless of the month and your income, so what you personally end up with varies. When you are employed by a company, however, you usually get steady pay, regardless of the business's monthly gross income. On the flip side of that, as an employer, you have to pay your employees, regardless of income, so you will be the one left out in the cold during a slim month.

Retail is notorious for this type of seasonal variation. If you always wanted to own your own clothing store, you will have to plan by the quarter rather than month by month. At first, such variation often inflicts heart palpitations on new business owners. After a while, you can learn to expect the down times, even if you don't ever like them.

Being organized and keeping financial records is a part of every business, yet those jobs frequently have nothing to do with the skills of the person who goes into business. Nevertheless, you need to start with the first lesson any business school student learns: business owners need a business plan. Yet, how many small business owners develop one before going into business? Very few, I suspect.

A business plan represents the profile of the work you've done to determine that your business could be viable—market research, projections of costs and income, profit and loss, and so on. The fact that you have constructed such a plan shows that you have thought through your business idea before going into business yourself or, at least, you've thought through the business aspects of the business. Many talented people think through the creative aspects of their businesses in great detail without ever considering the financial aspects. If you are looking for financing, though, no investor will consider talking with you unless you have a business plan. If numbers are not your forte, you can always get some help, but you do need a business plan.

Although owning your own business does mean that you're in charge, it definitely doesn't mean the end of those dreaded deadlines, and guess who will get blamed if you don't meet them? (Remember where the buck stops.) You need to be a very responsible, honest person to be successfully self-employed. If you try to place the blame on others, your reputation is likely to suffer fairly quickly, and customers can, and do, go other places where they will be treated with respect.

When Rolando, a wholesaler of truck parts, didn't meet the deadlines he had set with customers during the early days of his business, he would blame his supplier for not getting materials to him on time. He also blamed shippers for slow deliveries. After nine months, some of the other people involved with him began to shift their business to another wholesaler. When Rolando asked why they had left his business, one man told him that the word had gotten around that he blamed his delays on other people, and they didn't like that. Since they all did business with the same suppliers and transportation sources, and they did not have similar delay problems, Rolando's reputation as an honest businessman was ruined. He eventually had to go out of business.

When you are in business for yourself, pleasing clients is the name of the game. In fact, your clients are essentially your bosses when you are self-employed. If customers aren't happy, they won't come back, and soon you'll be out of business. You must please them—or else.

That is sometimes easier said than done. Dealing with the public can be the hardest job in the world. When you were in a big company, you were protected, in a sense. When you're self-employed, especially in a small business, the loss or displeasure of even one customer will cause a snag you don't need.

The reality of self-employment has its up and down sides. Weighing these against each other provides one guideline for you to decide whether or not to take the plunge. Much like parenting, it's impossible to realize what being your own boss is going to be like before you actually do it. It's probably just as well, too, or there might not be many self-employed people. Nevertheless, although the difficulty of the work load and the variety of challenges are impossible to imagine, truly independent people wouldn't have it any other way!

For you in particular, your drives, dreams, and personality will determine whether or not self-employment is a good idea for you. Now let's look at the impact of ADD on that decision.

Self-Employment and ADD

From my experience, it appears that a disproportionate number of people with ADD decide to go the self-employment route, compared to the population as a whole, and they are some of the happiest people who have ADD. They frequently open the types of businesses that use special skills or talents, as opposed to a business that takes "business sense" or that anyone could run if they wanted to be in business.

The special talent or creative interest of people who are ADD leads many to self-employment, because no one else can showcase that talent as well as the person who possesses it. Talented people usually know exactly how they'd like to do things, and it's difficult to fit such individualistic images into someone else's company.

When a creative person gets a new idea, he usually doesn't want to wait around for a committee or supervisor to decide, "Okay, you can move on it." Frequently, people who are creative are less concerned about making money or making a business successful than they are about plying their trade. So the creative ADD person often wants to "go for it," whether the talent is artistic, mechanical, or technical.

Outwardly Expressive ADD people tend to have the kind of entrepreneurial spirit that gets businesses started. They are often charismatic leaders who can get things going, and they use their hyperactive energy to initiate and start up the businesses.

Being bullheaded, like many people with Outwardly Expressive ADD are, can be an asset when you're heading up your own operation. This characteristic, which doesn't go over very well when you're an employee, creates the strong will useful for the self-employed person to possess. As one woman told me, "If my boss told me something I didn't agree with, I would think he was nuts. And I'd have gone ahead and done it my own way, which doesn't really lend itself to very high marks on an evaluation." She did much better when she worked for herself.

Someone with Highly Structured ADD, the perfectionist who pays attention to every detail, is controlling and wants things his own way. In many settings a liability, this trait can turn into an asset when he is working for himself. By softening his edges a little, especially when dealing with the public, and learning to be at least moderately accepting of other people's weaknesses, he can become a take-charge boss who masterminds his way to business success.

As I have mentioned, a greater proportion of people with ADD seems to have the drive to be self-employed than does that of the population as a whole. Many of us have an almost "missionary" zeal about our interests, which leads to an absolute need to work toward the goals we value. Anything else makes for unhappiness. I don't believe this drive is caused by failure to be able to make it in the corporate world; I think it's innate. Not only was it always there, but it never seems to go away. Even when we are successfully employed by others, with few headaches and great rewards, the dream to do our own thing persists.

Should You Try It?

No one can tell you whether self-employment is right for you—except you. You have to listen to your heart. If your heart sings when you think about going into business for yourself—if your heart feels tight or you feel trapped when you think about working for someone else—you have the first component necessary to go for self-employment.

To be sure, you must consider other factors, too, but I have learned that there are some of us who don't seem to have a choice about going into business for ourselves. We *have* to do it. Working at something that doesn't bring us joy creates so much stress that we can become sick and depressed. On the other hand, working at something that we love creates so much energy that we are determined to make a go of it. That determination is the key. I believe that anyone who really wants to be self-employed can be as successful at self-employment as he or she can be at any other job. It is just a matter of using your brains in conjunction with your heart and talents and not quitting as long as you *want* to do the work.

That doesn't mean that you can never return to being an employee. You may wish to try self-employment for a while to see how it feels. If it is not all you thought it would be, you can feel free to change your mind, or you may decide to change the type of self-employment. Always give yourself that freedom of choice. When you do, you can know that you are designing a life that you desire, not one in which you are a hapless victim of circumstances.

If you're just not sure whether you want to try self-employment, ask yourself these questions, and you might see your direction taking shape:

- If you are working for someone else what is your current emotional state?
- Do you desire to be self-employed? This is different from someone telling you that you ought to do it.
- In what stage of life are you? This includes the types of obligations you have—financial, family, and other commitments.
- Are you a responsible person?
- Do you mind hard work?
- Have you built up your work skills sufficiently that you can go it alone without supervision?
- Do you know anything about running a business—yours or anyone else's?
- Have you gained experience in the field in which you are interested by working for someone else, learning what the business would be like?
- What kind of support, financial and emotional, do you have to start your business?

- What is the worst that would happen if you went into business for yourself, and are you willing to take that risk?

- What would you do if the worst happened?

- Can you imagine not being in business for yourself?

There are certainly no right or wrong answers to these questions, but if you are even considering opening your own business, these are questions you need to answer for yourself, maybe even questions you need to wrestle with a bit.

Let's say you've given this whole matter a lot of thought, weighed the pros and cons, and decided to give self-employment a try. You envision, design, and start your business. Now it is up and running. What then? Is it the kind of business you would like to continue working with, or do you now have to administrate a business that no longer requires creative input—the business aspect that attracted you in the first place?

One of the biggest problems faced by people who are ADD comes from the difference between creating a business, a creative act, and running a business, an administrative act. The creative aspect of business development helps a person with ADD stay focused and interested, while administering a business is often experienced as boring and difficult. Building something new is exciting. Keeping something going is not—at least, most creative people with ADD don't think so.

So what are the options you may want to consider? You may even want to make them a part of an original business plan. For one thing, you could always sell the business. Otherwise, you could take on a partner and turn the running of the business over to that person. It's a great idea to consider these options ahead of time. To be perfectly honest, I never thought of those issues in advance because I was so wrapped up in what I was creating. (Now you know part of the reason why I have had many business successes *and* a lot of failure.) If you want to save yourself lots of trouble, make a business plan with an "ejection seat" designed in ahead of time.

You may wish to cultivate someone else to take over your business. You might set it up with a buy-in capability for employees. You might also consider enrolling in a business class. Even if the class itself does not interest you, this is a good place to meet people who are also interested in self-employment—and might make good future partners for you.

Whatever direction you take, it is very important to give yourself permission to leave the business when you've gotten it up and running. In our culture the tendency exists to feel that you have to stay with something forever. Most people call that responsibility. I challenge that concept, however, and ask you to realize that having opened a business and carried it to some level of success can be a meaningful completion of your involvement. It's all right to let it go then, preferably with as much gain as possible.

Suppose you try opening your own business, but you don't make it. Several important lessons can be learned from being a part of an unsuccessful business. First of all, it doesn't necessarily mean that you are inadequate or a failure. Having been there myself, I know you probably feel that way, but it's not true.

Think of your experience as a learning opportunity. Look at what you did well and what you didn't. Then, once you've recovered from the pain of having had a business failure, consider whether you still like the idea of being self-employed. If you do, make use of what you learned from the previous experience.

Maybe, like Tyrone, you failed to include a structured person on your payroll. When Tyrone decided to open his body shop, he was sure he could be a big success. He had good skills, loved people, and wanted to provide a fair service to his customers. What Tyrone didn't do was get someone to set up the books right away. Instead, he carried pieces of paper around in his pockets. He made notes on a pad, which he promised himself he'd turn into records as soon as he had time, though he really didn't know when that would be or what he would have to do.

As you can guess, Tyrone never found that extra time. There were always new ideas to pursue and new customers to serve. Occasionally, when he did stop working, he was exhausted and couldn't think anymore. Besides, he didn't know where to start.

After a few months the whole paperwork end of his business was totally out of control. He had no figures to give the IRS and had made no tax deposits. He had no reserves because he'd sunk all his money back into the business buying equipment, and he had done a lot of work on credit for people. Sadly, Tyrone learned that not every customer is grateful for a job well done; neither do all people pay their bills.

In less than a year, Tyrone's business went under.

Five years later, newly married Tyrone tried again. He just couldn't stand to work for someone else. More importantly, his wife was a bookkeeper and wanted to work with him in the business. She believed in him *and* knew his inadequacies. From the day the business opened, she kept track of everything. Their teamwork quickly built the business that Tyrone had always dreamed of.

Ilsa having accumulated five years' experience after receiving her master's degree in counseling, decided she wanted to go into private practice. She too was skillful, but unlike Tyrone, she knew how to start and maintain such a business and felt she had good connections.

Through no fault of hers, though, the mental health scene had begun a downward turn. The public was disenchanted with the many programs that discharged patients, whether they had received the help they needed or not, when their insurance money ran out. Also, managed health care was beginning to take over, limiting the choices of mental health providers for many people, and adding reams of paperwork.

Where Ilsa previously could have covered her expenses and made a fair income, there were now not enough hours in the day to accumulate the income she needed. After two years of struggling, Ilsa called it quits and went back to work for a company in a related field. She had done nothing wrong; the timing was just wrong for what she had to offer.

Though for a while both Tyrone and Ilsa felt as if their worlds had come to an end, they both took stock and figured out what was wrong. Ilsa understood that she was in a grief reaction for having lost her dream. Although Tyrone didn't think of it that way, he lived through his grief and was ready to try again.

If you experience failure, ask yourself why it happened, but be kind to yourself, because you are grieving from the loss of a dream. Do whatever you need to do to recover, financially and emotionally, then reconsider whether you still like the idea of self-employment. If you do, use what you learned and try again. If you don't want to try again, that's fine, too.

Remember, *you* get to design your own life, and self-employment is not for everyone.

What Happens If You Don't Give Self-Employment a Try?

If you are really a candidate for self-employment—that is, if it's in your blood—you are likely to experience depression or lack of success on other jobs if you don't take the plunge.

Many people want to be self-employed but never try it out because of the objections of their spouses. I've never been able to get Morris out of my mind. At forty-something, Morris's depression was extensive. It had, in fact, become a way of life. He and his wife came to me for marriage counseling after he had been unemployed for a year and a half, after having lost another in a long succession of jobs. It seemed as if his work was mediocre, and he was one of the first employees to be let go when things got tight.

In the process of trying to discover what his chronic job situation was about, I asked him in private what he would like to do if he had a magic wand and could do anything he wanted and be sure of success. For the first time his face lit up, and he said, "Have my own landscape business." I asked him if he'd talked with his wife about it and he said, "Oh, yes, and she'd kill me if I ever mentioned it again. I need to do something responsible."

It turned out that his wife was petrified of the idea of his being self-employed. She nagged him endlessly and anxiously about getting a *real* job. She was angry about his failures. She would neither entertain any possibility that he needed to pursue his dream, nor would she stop nagging him to do something that obviously didn't fit him. The last time I saw them, Morris was still depressed, and his wife was still nagging.

Many people do eventually go into business for themselves, but do it later in life. Women frequently fall into this pattern, putting off pursuing adventure and dreams until the kids are grown. Some very successful enterprises come about this way. One woman I know started a swimsuit company at age fifty, designing suits for the less-than-wonderful figure. Her youngest child was securely on her own, her husband was supportive, and she simply couldn't imagine continuing to do what she'd done for the last twenty years.

When she shyly told her husband her idea, to her surprise he said, "Go for it!" This woman's familiarity with her ADD and the problems it sometimes caused made her fearful of trying to run a business. Thanks to help from several of her husband's business contacts, however, she found the support she needed, and she designed her way to considerable success.

Some people who don't have that kind of support make the leap to self-employment anyway. Trudy is a case in point. At first, Trudy's divorce sent her reeling. What was she going to do? At fifty-five, her life seemed like a total failure. Her kids didn't think she was great, her ex thought she was useless, and her parents thought she must have done some pretty terrible things to have created such a mess. On top of that, Trudy had almost no money and no real professional training or job skills of any substance.

Eating a sundae with a friend on a Friday evening, bemoaning her fate, she made the comment, "If I'd have known how my life was going to turn out, I'd have gone ahead at twenty writing romance novels, and to heck with what people thought." Her friend almost flippantly said, "So why not do it now? What do you have to lose?"

For a minute, Trudy started to discount the remark, but something rang true in it for her. She heard a voice in her head saying, Why not? So she went for it. During the days she worked temporary jobs to earn just enough money to cover modest expenses. The rest of the time, she wrote and wrote and wrote. She found that she could make trades with someone from a local writer's group to edit her work. With her ADD, Trudy's downfall had been her punctuation, but never her imagination.

Trudy had talent. With some assistance from her mentor, she was able to make her first sale. As a result, she felt motivated, hopeful, and valuable.

Sometimes, in retirement people find that they have opportunities for second careers. Often these careers turn out to be forays into self-employment. What a great way to use the money provided through the buy-out packages offered by many companies for early retirement. Talk about a new lease on life!

How to Keep the Money You Make

Keeping the money you make is the kind of problem that people laugh about, saying, "Boy, I sure wish I had that kind of problem." But it's no laughing matter, and people with ADD often have trouble hanging onto money. This can be an especially difficult issue for people who are self-employed.

Several ADD characteristics contribute to this problem. For one thing, the compassionate, empathetic parts of us often want to play philanthropist. However, not being very good about keeping track of money, we may not know how much to give away or when to give it. Planning ahead for lean times when infrequent expenses arise may not come to mind at the moment that the impulse to be generous strikes.

Gretchen was a successful owner of a dress shop whose income varied greatly with the seasons. When her income level was high, she tended to make presents to the people she loved as well as to those who happened to cross her path with special needs.

Gretchen knew how much she had made, but two problems caused her to have trouble keeping the money under control. First, she didn't know how to plan for the irregular payments that needed to be made, such as property taxes or quarterly medical-insurance payments. She knew they would be coming up, but somehow she couldn't figure out where to put the money on a regular basis, separate from her monthly living-expense money. She did think about opening another bank account, but she already had trouble keeping up with the one she had. Somehow, that didn't seem like it would really help her keep control of the insurance and tax monies.

Second, Gretchen's creative mind had already spent that income twenty different ways. Any one of the twenty would have left enough for practical things, but in her thoughts she wasn't able to sort one spending path from the other nineteen. So she just sort of jumped into this mental muddle and gave a little bit here and a little bit there. Before she knew it, most of her income was gone.

Impulsive spending is another problem for people with ADD. The high that comes from buying something new seems wonderful, an increase in the very chemicals in the brain needed to focus attention, and provides a grand relief from the boredom that often surrounds mundane living. Unfortunately, though, the high doesn't last. So, no matter what the purchase, it eventually becomes just another consumable item, even if it remains around the house for years; the luster can wear off quickly.

Plowing the money you make back into your business can create the illusion that you are being sensible. However, it is all too easy to create a business with high expenses and low net gain. Before you know it, you are supporting a lot of other people or working a lot of hours for very little gain.

Jack was a business owner with ADD who hated to make extra money. He had no clue what to do with it. It burned a hole in his pocket, he spent it, and his wife got real sore with him. That was a scenario that repeated itself over and over again.

Jack loved gadgets and simply couldn't resist buying whatever the latest model was when it first came on the market. Of course, that's when the item would be at its highest price. Then he'd run out of money, and his family would pinch pennies until the next flow of money arrived and the next impulsive purchase occurred. Jack's addiction to the high he obtained making gadget purchases eventually cost him his marriage.

One woman I know frankly confesses that her addiction is to creativity and new ideas. "I get my charge out of them, so that is where my time and money go. It's not a lot different from buying all the supplies for a new craft but never making the item," she says. "I start creating a new enterprise in my mind, spend time buying supplies for it, experiment with developing it, pay someone to consult about it, and then—when it would be time to take that next step, the one that would mean getting down to actually working on the business plan or production—I'm low on funds, and I lose interest. Off I go onto some new idea that pops into my head. My resume looks like a kaleidoscope of interests. Maybe someday I'll learn to weave them together. What a great idea!"

Many people with ADD, including many business owners, experience terror when trying to deal with money. Though they are willing to try to track their funds better and are disciplined about the work they do, they are not able to carry this discipline over into money management. It simply eludes them, and neither they nor any accountant can say why.

If this is your case, your best bet is to get a money manager or accountant who can set up a *very* simple system for you and your business. Others may talk about all the money that can be made by this or that investment, but I promise you, the difficulty of trying to keep track of your money in high-yield investments may end up costing you money. High finance is a different world that speaks a different language, and there's no money management/ADD dictionary around that can help you translate.

Make your accountant your best friend, figuratively speaking. Have him or her put you on a salary, even though all the money is actually yours. Have the accountant plan for the irregular expenses and put something away for the unexpected. With the rest, invest in something that does not take your continual attention and understanding to track. The trick is to trust your accountant and stick to the plan the two of you develop. I'm not suggesting that you trust just *any* accountant, but trust your feelings about the person you are considering, and keep track of those feelings.

One bad experience I had occurred because I didn't listen to my gut-level feeling. I hid, as so many of us do, from confronting the accountant because I *felt* something was wrong. Because I didn't have a clue what it might be or how to find it, however, I just let the situation continue until it came to an abrupt halt—with me out many thousands of dollars.

In retrospect, I could have hired a second accountant to look at what the first accountant was doing. At the time, I might have considered that a foolish expense. In the end, though, it would have saved me a lot of money. As insecure as I was about money, I kept quiet and hoped the whole thing would go away. I hope you can learn from my experience; I know I have. Trust your gut level feelings.

Teaming Up: Two Heads Are Better Than One

Two school friends decided to take a fling after graduating from college. Both loved the outdoors and wanted to travel, but they needed money to do it. So they decided to start a company called Adventures. At first their money-making schemes were far-fetched, pie-in-the-sky fantasies, especially the ideas that Ed came up with.

Ed, who is ADD, had majored in communications in college. He liked to write but was pretty undisciplined, barely meeting deadlines, and his work needed some good editing. What he liked even better was talking, so he took a lot of speech and broadcast classes.

Randy also loved the outdoors but was more quiet. His biology major fit his interest in native plants all over the world. He had good writing skills, though most of his articles and papers were strictly factual. When he and Ed brainstormed, he was the one taking notes and organizing their ideas.

In two months they mapped out a plan of traveling around the world for two years. They would pursue Randy's interest in native plants. Randy would write articles for submission to magazines, while Ed would make contacts for giving talks and act as the publicist for Randy's work.

Ed also contacted an uncle of his in the import-export business. They decided Ed could act as a buyer for exotic seeds and bulbs from the countries they planned to visit. It sounded exciting to Ed, and it would give them a small flow of steady income.

Not only did the two men have a wonderful time traveling, they ended up with a company that booked presentations all around the world. They continued to pool their interests and skills, and the company became very successful.

Ed benefited from the organizational skills that Randy brought to their travels and their almost constant brainstorming. Randy helped Ed think through the many wild schemes that came to his mind and make decisions that would be in Ed's best interest. Also, Randy loved the excitement that Ed brought to their partnership; it kept him from involving himself only in the sometimes tedious work of plant identification and classification. Ed also had great ideas that Randy never thought of but which he could certainly use.

Because of Ed, Randy eventually finished a doctorate degree. That way Ed could advertise their tours under the name of Dr. Randy Conan, internationally known biologist. They figured that would make their talks more valuable and create a larger audience. It worked!

Teamwork, either as employed coworkers or self-employed partners, makes all the difference for people with ADD and for people who
are not ADD. Each benefits from the other, and, frankly, they are of
equal value to one another. ADD is truly an asset!

10

If You Don't Have ADD

When you're not ADD, working with someone who is ADD is challenging. I give you a lot of credit for caring enough to learn about this very special way of being wired. Then again, you may be paying attention for your own survival.

As you learn about ADD, you will be rewarded by finding easier ways to work with those of us who have ADD, and you will become aware of the assets that we do bring to the table. We need you, and you can benefit from us. It's all in the teaming. Together we make a whole that is hard to beat.

Though not always easy, it's usually quite interesting working with people who are ADD. You'll discover that ADD affects every aspect of work life—the tangible areas such as productivity, organization, and quality control, and the emotional elements that affect relationships, mood, and attitude.

All job performance ultimately depends on productivity, whether we're talking about how many gadgets come off the assembly line, how many sales are made, or how much time it takes to dig the right-shaped ditch in which to lay pipe. When a worker falls short, the project suffers. People who have faulty work habits or inadequate work skills create a shortfall that means others have to pick up the slack—people like you.

People with ADD often seem to have more potential than they are using on the job. That discrepancy creates a gap, and you may be the one who has to make up the difference to fill in that gap or see that the difference is made up.

Does that mean you are working with someone who is lazy, doesn't care, or ought to be fired? Probably not. It does mean, however, that production is compromised because your coworker is so easily distracted. Staying on task to reach a goal is one of the greatest difficulties a person with ADD faces.

Perhaps your ADD coworker found it easier to talk her way into a job than to follow through with assignments. Maybe her ideas are creative and promising, but when it comes to production, she falls down on the job. Is she energetic at the beginning of a project, but winds up needing you to pick up the pieces she cannot complete? That would be very frustrating for you. Maybe her production is high at one time and crashes at another. Uneven work performance is another attribute of ADD. You never know what to expect.

Organizational difficulties, whether it's organization of time, projects, or tools, are among the worst workplace problems for people who are ADD. You may not be able to imagine the jumble that occurs in the mind of someone with ADD, because you are dealing with a mind that simply processes information in a different way from yours. Yes, you might misplace papers yourself once in a while or occasionally be late on an assignment. For your ADD coworkers, though, organizational difficulties create daily, or even hourly, crises—not a once in awhile problem.

Yet, people with ADD do have their own organizational systems. They're just very, very different from yours. Older workers, who have lived long enough to discover and use it effectively, have an advantage. Younger workers with ADD might not yet have discovered their organizational system.

The on-off switch inside people with ADD works to make them late starting things and, once started, slow at being able to stop. There seems to be no dimmer switch that allows your ADD coworkers to shift gears. Rather than smoothly oiled work machines, they may appear to be sputtering and puttering trying to get going, or they may also appear to be relics that don't know when to quit.

Perfectionism is another aspect of inefficient work habits. Not all people with ADD are perfectionists, but many people who have a lot of Highly Structured ADD are. So often I've heard, "I don't even want to start that project, because I know what it means: I'll be doing it forever, never satisfied with the end results." Driven by an internal pressure, this type of person simply cannot respond to the work pace of those around him. It's not that he doesn't want to—he just can't, at least not without a major effort.

On the other hand, many people with ADD who have trouble starting a project, feel a letdown after the excitement of cutting the deal that created the project. They were excited and stimulated by the project design and negotiations, but actually producing the work bores them, so they put it off. At other times, your ADD coworker delays the beginning of a project because she cannot figure out which step needs to be done first or which materials to gather. These are organizational issues again.

One aspect of delaying to start projects, though, has a positive force behind it: people with ADD are better able to focus attention when under pressure. Consequently, putting something off until the last minute creates the pressure needed to go full force and get the job done.

Whether you're working with or for someone with any of these ADD attributes, you can see how your life will be affected. Faced with a style of work that is drastically different from your own, and one that you may not understand, can be quite frustrating. Understanding that the person doesn't intend to cause problems for you may help.

Emotionally, ADD leaves its marks, too. A strong possibility exists that if you are working with someone who is extremely sensitive, so much so that you feel you must walk on eggshells, you may be dealing with someone who is ADD. Perhaps your colleague or coworker is a hot-head who makes you feel as if you were walking in a mine field. Then again, you may be faced with a coworker who never seems to think before speaking or taking impulsive actions.

If your coworker is sensitive, impulsive, moody, or hot-tempered, ADD may be the culprit that is disrupting your work situation. Each of these attributes can be quite unsettling, but they do not mean your coworker is a bad person. Nor does it mean all is lost, though time and effort often must be spent by everyone involved to repair the damage.

Even more frustrating than a coworker who is disorganized or impulsive is one who appears lazy or dishonest. You have every right to feel unwilling to put up with such behavior, but you do need to be sure that what you're looking at is actually laziness or dishonesty, not an inability to concentrate or a near-fatal lack of organization.

When Candice told her supervisor that she had left her reports at home, she was lying (chapter four). She was not a hardened criminal. Instead, she was a frightened woman with ADD who very much wanted to complete her reports and do the job she was assigned. Her intent was honorable; it was her behavior that was dishonest. Candice may even have thought that she could finish all of her reports if she worked all night. You might think that's completely unrealistic, but Candice might not have realized that her sense of time and her ability to break long-term projects down into small segments is significantly impaired.

Fear, shame, and guilt are frequent companions of people with ADD. If your coworker has ADD but doesn't know it, he is probably just as irritated with himself as you are. Knowing this may help you realize that surface appearances may not be what they seem. That doesn't, however, mean you should simply accept inadequate performance. It does mean you can add understanding to the limits you set.

Your Reactions to Working with Someone Who Has ADD

When your coworker failed to complete her part of a project on time so that you could finish yours, you probably felt irritated or even angry—especially if the boss jumped on you for not getting your work in on time. Remember the time you had to redo everything your partner gave you because it was so poorly organized? How about the time your new employee, who looked so good on paper, turned out to be unable to produce a simple, clearly written summary of the first quarter's work? And what about the time your boss pressured you to get a job done but didn't give you the information you needed until the last minute?

On a practical level, saying that there was an interruption of work flow would be an understatement. A workplace in which these extremes are common—either sitting with nothing to do or frantically working overtime—is not a sane work environment. Also, because most work settings require teamwork, when one cog is out of step, you, your work, and the whole project suffer.

When you pay the price because a coworker with ADD created a bottleneck, no one expects you to be pleased. In fact, anger would be a pretty normal reaction. Frustration, fear of being unable to perform up to par yourself, and feelings of helplessness may all sweep through you. Each results from something happening that you feel you have no power to do anything about.

When things start to go wrong in the workplace, the first thing you are likely to feel is confusion. You realize things are not going the way you expected, but you can't quite figure out what's gone wrong. Your specific reaction will depend on whether you tend to blame others for things that happen or blame yourself. You'll either look around outside yourself for the cause of the problem or look at yourself. One way or the other, you'll begin to feel stressed.

Have you ever found yourself getting depressed, obsessing about work *after* work, talking to your spouse or friends and wondering whether it's time for you to move on to a new job? You may find yourself not feeling very well, being fatigued or even depressed, unable to sleep soundly, or losing your taste for the pleasures of life that you usually enjoy. These are all sure signs that you are under stress and something is wrong.

I am not trying to say that every disturbance or depression that affects any employee is caused by a coworker who has ADD. That would be ridiculous. Yet, there are times when an ADD coworker does cause problems like this, and neither you nor your coworker really knows what to do about it.

The key is that you can learn how to deal with it. The first step is to establish the intent of the other person's behavior—or lack of intent—rather than making assumptions. Please do not assume that the person is purposely doing whatever he or she is doing, doesn't care, or that the behavior is aimed at you.

For example, when Gladys, a hairdresser, failed to show up on time for work, Margaret, the shop owner, decided she had had enough. Late for work one more time, she thought. I guess Gladys doesn't care about her job. If she did, she'd get here on time. Margaret was basing her assumption on how she would behave if she cared about a job and wanted to keep it.

Fortunately, Margaret took Gladys aside and said, "Hey, what's going on here? You were late again, the third time this week." Then she asked, rather than told, Gladys, "Don't you care about your job?"

Gladys broke into tears. "Of course I care about my job," she said. "I love working here." Margaret, who was rarely late for any appointment, felt confused. In her mind, she couldn't make the connection between Gladys's liking her job and being late. She also realized, though, that Gladys seemed to thoroughly enjoy her customers, seemed happy while at work, often stayed late to help out, and was always very apologetic about being late.

So Margaret softened her tone and asked, "Then why are you late so often? It makes me nervous having customers waiting, and it's bad for the shop's reputation."

Gladys, crying but feeling relieved, explained how hard she was trying to get to work on time. She had always had trouble getting places on time, but she thought she'd outgrow it. It didn't seem to matter whether she wanted to be on time or not: things just happened. She could manage being on time for one or two days, but then, as she relaxed a bit, things just got in the way, or she would sleep through her alarm clock. And she said her brain didn't seem to wake up in the morning until after she'd been up for a couple of hours.

Having identified the problem, Margaret suggested that Gladys could start work an hour later and work through lunch, and she'd still get up at the same time. Since one of the problems was Gladys's getting distracted and puttering around her apartment, Margaret volunteered to call Gladys when it was time for her to leave for work. Gladys promised to leave then, no matter what she was doing.

With the support of Margaret, someone who cared and felt Gladys was a valuable employee, most of the problem was resolved. Gladys eventually became used to her schedule, and after a while she no longer needed that reminder call from Margaret.

Being chronically late to appointments is a problem that plagues many people with ADD. Some who choose to use medication find that if they set an alarm forty-five minutes to an hour before they need to get up, take their medication, reset the alarm, go back to sleep, then wake up to their alarm a second time, they get up much easier, more clear-headed, and awake.

When Eduardo failed to get his expense reports in on time, Sherry was unable to complete her reports for the boss. Because Eduardo complained constantly about having to do the reports, she thought he was purposely not turning them in. She couldn't figure out why he was being so obstinate.

What Sherry didn't know was that Eduardo *couldn't* do his reports. Each time he tried, he came up with different figures. His head would ache, and he seemed to be able to find only half of his receipts at any time.

His complaining about having to do the reports was a cover-up for not being able to do them, but Sherry didn't realize this until she confronted him rather angrily, "I don't care whether you want to do these or not—I'm sick and tired of being late with my reports because of you. Get them to me on time, or I'll have to tell the boss that you're the reason my work is always late."

Eduardo was embarrassed, but he told Sherry the truth. Once she understood, she made a deal with him to do the reports for him. All Eduardo had to do was put every receipt he got into an envelope and give them to her weekly, along with his mileage figures. The problem was solved. Sherry didn't really mind doing the reports because that type of work was easy for her. Sherry was no longer mad at Eduardo, and Eduardo could concentrate on what he excelled at, selling.

It is always possible to reach a solution when the true issues of a problem are understood.

When you find yourself getting extremely angry at work, stop what you're doing. Leave as soon as you can. Talk your feelings through with someone other than the person who has angered you, someone who will not gossip about what you are saying. Your intent in talking about your feelings should not be to tell tales but to discharge enough emotion to be able to think clearly again, so you can switch into a problem-solving mode.

Find out why you feel threatened by the other person's actions or words. Anger is always a cover-up emotion, which means that another emotion lies under it. Anger is present to protect some vulnerable part of you—a part that feels afraid, helpless, hopeless, or frustrated. Once you've determined what underlies your anger, you can begin to understand more about yourself.

Sherry realized that the underlying cause of her anger was her fear that her boss would think she was not doing a good job. At that point, she was ready either to make her demands of Eduardo or, if he didn't produce, to tell her boss the truth to protect herself and what she needed, her job.

Once you've understood the cause of your anger, fear, or frustration, you can formulate a plan to deal with it. Clear-headed, free of assumptions and judgments, you can find out the other person's intent simply by asking, for example, "I need to know why I'm not getting your reports on time." Or, "When you blurt things out in the meetings, I feel embarrassed and out of control. I need to know how you see what's happening." Don't accuse the other person; just ask him to explain how he sees the issue.

Of course, if the person with ADD fails to provide you with information or accuses you in return, you'll have to use another tactic. When Frank's boss tried to talk with him about why an order was not filled (chapter two) and Frank stalked off, his boss was left in a difficult situation. When the boss tried again after lunch to talk to Frank to no avail, his hands were tied: if Frank hadn't quit, his boss would have had to be confrontational with him, probably handing him an ultimatum.

If an ADD coworker or employee, or anyone for that matter, won't talk with you about a problem, then an impasse is reached, and you will have to decide how to go around the person. Even though you may know that fear underlies the person's inability or unwillingness to talk with you, business is business. Your responsibility to help the other person solve the problem goes only so far, and there's only so much you can be expected to do.

Your Working Relationship with the Subordinate Who Has ADD

If you're the boss and your employee is ADD—or you think he or she is ADD—it's important to find ways to use those ADD traits in a positive manner. By helping bring out the positives, you are not only helping your coworkers, you might even be saving their jobs. If they have skills and talents that you like and that are useful to you, then you will want to work with them. If not, you need to know how to counsel them into a job that fits them better.

No one expects you to diagnose ADD in an employee or coworker; that isn't something you are qualified to do. I do want you to be familiar with the signs and symptoms that indicate a person may be ADD, however, so that you will know how to work with the ADD-like symptoms. Following are four checklists to help you decide whether your employee or coworker needs your help and in what areas.

These characteristics indicate the possibility of problems with concentration and attention:

_____ Has trouble completing assignments or jobs without getting distracted
_____ Seems to daydream a lot
_____ Has trouble reading because his mind wanders
_____ Jumps from one thing to another, barely finishing anything
_____ Hates being interrupted, finding it hard to get back on task
_____ Isolates himself away from other people, totally concentrating on what he is doing

These items tend to indicate the kinds of problems people with ADD have in the organizational area:

_____ Has difficulty getting or staying organized
_____ Works with piles of paper that get higher and higher

_____ Can't find papers that are filed

_____ Has trouble keeping track of tools or implements used for work

_____ Finds it hard to break tasks down into manageable bits

_____ Is often late or unaware of time

_____ Tends to take on more than can be done in a reasonable amount of time

_____ Is a perfectionist with a detailed organizational system

_____ Gets very upset when his organization is interfered with

When a person is well disciplined, he may appear organized on the surface but feel very unorganized. He may also cover this inadequacy by having a great secretary or administrative assistant or by constantly creating new, innovative projects, although never following through on them.

The following items have to do with the hypersensitivity experienced by people who are ADD:

_____ Is supersensitive to criticism

_____ Is easily distracted by noise, complains of smells, or reacts to the environment, including the covering of the office furniture

_____ Is extremely empathetic, becoming overly emotionally involved with interpersonal issues in the workplace

_____ Gets very angry or upset over "little" things

_____ Reacts strenuously in relation to the underdog

_____ Cries, becomes angry easily, or has large mood swings in response to workplace issues

_____ Is hypercritical of others or self

Impulsivity, impatience, and hyperactivity, such as are manifested in the following, are characteristics shared by people with ADD:

_____ Is rarely physically still

_____ Has a high level of energy, appearing to be a whirlwind who is accomplishing a lot, but crashing to a standstill when stopping

_____ Is restless, paces, subtly moves a lot, or hates being confined inside a building or confined to a desk

_____ Rarely moves, exhibiting hyperactivity; rigidly sedentary

_____ Speaks without thinking

_____ Acts without thinking

_____ Seems very impulsive, with no thought for the outcome of his actions or words

_____ Is impatient, unable to wait without complaining

_____ Hates lines, being put on hold, or not being able to get rapid results

A person who is well socialized has learned to mask these despite feeling them inside.

If your employee or coworker has a lot of these characteristics, you would do well to implement ADD-compensating adjustments that will make his life, and your life, better. It doesn't really matter whether or not he actually has ADD; you don't need a definitive diagnosis before making some adjustments to make life easier in the workplace. And don't be fooled by an employee who has a lot of talent or skill in one area or who is very bright. That person may still be ADD, and problems will show up as soon as the person is working outside his area of expertise.

So, the popular talk show host who has trouble keeping track of her tapes or logging her public service announcements may be ADD. The hotheaded mechanic who can fix anything, anywhere, anytime but can't pass the state licensing exam may be ADD. The soldier who was successful in the military but fell apart trying to hold down an unstructured civilian job also might have ADD.

Once you've identified that your employee or coworker might be ADD, you can initiate a conversation on the topic and provide a mini-education about how people are wired differently. Just let the person know that many people who have trouble with organization, sitting still, or being impulsive turn out to be ADD. You might want to suggest that the person check into that possibility. Furthermore, let her know that you are willing to help her work with these issues to improve the work environment for everyone, if she is willing.

You could say, "You and I seem to work differently. Let me tell you what I see, and then I'd like to know how you see our situation. I'd like to tell you what I need and find out what you need. I think that will be helpful for both of us."

With this kind of introduction, you don't have to say, "I think you have ADD." Instead, you can talk directly about the behaviors or attributes of ADD without mentioning ADD. Also, it's always a good idea to talk about the person's strengths. For example, you can say, "You're very talented, and by working on _____ you can make much more effective use of your talent." Remember, your job is to enlist the trust of the person so she will tell you what is needed to be a more effective worker.

If you are a boss with an ADD employee, working with her to accommodate her differences is not unlike working with any other employee to do the same. A boss's job is to maximize the strengths of the employee and minimize, or preferably strengthen, the weaknesses. That way you develop an effective team that gets the job done.

I would suggest setting up a regular "training" time for you and your employee to work together on this self-improvement project. You can learn more about ADD and ADD-like behavior by calling in a consultant to provide some training, if your company does that sort of thing. You can find out whether your area has an ADD support, education, or training group for you and your employee to attend. You can read up on ADD. If your employee or coworker does have a professional evaluation, ask whether she would allow a copy of the results and recommendations to be sent to you. That way you would better know how you can be helpful.

If the person is unwilling to work with you, then you may need to set a limit, saying, "Your work in the area of _____ is not acceptable, and it really has to be improved. If you choose not to work with me, that's okay, but you must get the job done. Otherwise, it's not in either of our best interests to work together."

If it is your coworker who is ADD or seems to be ADD, you have to be clear about what you are and are not willing to put up with. Your first job is to open the lines of communication between the two of you about the ADD-like characteristics that are showing up in your work together.

For example, Gwen and Calvin worked together in a music store. Calvin was a music teacher, and Gwen was in charge of inventory and retail sales. When Gwen noticed that Calvin was continually getting his schedule messed up, she decided to talk to him about it.

"Calvin, you are such a good teacher, but you seem to be having trouble keeping track of your schedule. What's up?" she asked.

When Calvin hemmed and hawed and looked uncomfortable, Gwen jumped in and said, "Would it be useful to you if I tried to help you figure out a system that might work better than the one you're using?"

Calvin was relieved and said it would be helpful. It took some time for them to get things running smoothly, but eventually they did. The words *attention deficit disorder* were never mentioned, even though it was later discovered that Calvin did have ADD.

Calvin and Gwen color-coded a weekly schedule, with one color for his in-store lessons and other colors for his paperwork time and off-site teaching. By setting the schedule by the door of the teaching room, Calvin had to walk by it and was able to check people in and out when they came for their lessons. There was a telephone there, too, so he could call home and leave himself a message about the time he needed to be somewhere the next day. Finally, he set up a small desk nearby at which he added up the hours he worked each day, leaving a duplicate report for Gwen. If he was away from the store at the end of the day, he would come in early the next morning and write this report first thing.

At first, Gwen helped him get into the habit of keeping track of things. Then she slowly turned the job over to him. Calvin told her how grateful he was for her help.

If you think Gwen went over and above the call of duty, and that you would not be willing to put that much time and effort into helping a coworker, don't feel guilty. This type of help is voluntary, not a requirement. Set your limits anywhere you want, and for heaven's sake, don't agree to anything that you don't want to do.

Feel free to support the other person without doing the job for him.

Consider coworkers Samuel and Walker. Walker was hyperactive, always thumping his foot, jiggling the table, drumming his fingers, and bouncing up and down. Samuel let Walker know that he understood Walker's need to move around a lot but that it made him nuts. Without blaming Walker, Samuel told him that he himself needed help because he wasn't getting any work done, and that one of them had to move his desk. They were able to talk together and decide which one could move easier. The other helped in the moving process. No blame. No shame. But there was change.

If Your Boss Is ADD

If it is your boss who is ADD, you need to be explicit when you deal with her or him. Before you talk with your boss about any ADD-trait problems, be prepared. Don't make an appointment with your boss and spend the time complaining. Instead, know what you want, the time frame in which you need it, and in what form you want it. Be clear that your ultimate goal is to support your boss's goals in the best way possible.

For example, Giselle's boss, Lila, a highly creative clothing designer, is an energetic entrepreneur who flies from one project to another, rarely finishing anything. Giselle is responsible for making all the preparations for the style shows and public displays showcasing Lila's new lines of clothing. Prior to every show, Lila must make certain decisions that only she can make. Giselle learned early on that pinning Lila down was quite tricky. When Giselle gave her several things to do at once, Lila didn't get back to her on any of them. Giselle then requested regular weekly meetings with Lila. At each meeting she gives Lila a typed copy of her requests, honed down to as few words as possible, and she keeps a copy for herself. After each request is a blank line to write Lila's answers. Giselle verbally introduces one question at a time, gives Lila a short time to decide on an answer, writes down the answer, then goes on to the next question. She has learned to keep the meetings short. If necessary, she schedules a second meeting during the week to keep Lila's attention fresh.

Never patronizing and always keeping an even tone of voice, Giselle manages to calm Lila down enough to be moderately effective in the meetings. When Lila gets off track, Giselle says, "Lila, I need an answer to this question. I'm making a note of this new concept you began to talk about. We can get back to it later, and the idea won't be lost, but now I need you to tell me your answer."

Lila appreciates Giselle, and Giselle admires Lila's talent. Together they have developed a dynamic team, and a close friendship is being built—all based on mutual respect—but it was originally up to Giselle to set limits on Lila. She made it clear that she needed to set those limits in order to support her boss's goals well.

When Carrie needed her boss to give her an okay on a topic for the magazine they were putting out, she said, "Look, we need to have a full staff meeting once a month to explain the editorial focus of the issue we're working on at that time. Without it, I am repeating myself twenty times, which wastes your time and money." Then she asked a direct question of her boss: "Will you give me an okay to call the meeting monthly so I can go over the plans for the issue we're working on?"

Notice that Carrie repeated her request in the form of a question. That way, if her boss, who she knew was easily distracted, had tuned out in the beginning, he had a chance to recoup without having to admit that he hadn't really been listening attentively. When she started the question, "Will you give me an okay," he realized that he would need to make a response, so he tuned in.

Carrie did not take his tuning out personally. She realized that was just how he was. He let her know in other ways that he appreciated her, and he truly did, both for her skills and for her kindness.

I do a lot of public speaking, and I have an agent who books those engagements for me. She recently said to me, "Lynn, just give me the names of the contacts you made at the conference. You don't need to take the time to type them out; just read them off to me over the phone. I realize keeping track of them is not your cup of tea, but I need them."

I thought, "Whew. She understands." So I read her names off scraps of paper, business cards, and a list I'd acquired somewhere. The job was done as painlessly as possible for both of us.

The professional employee takes responsibility for presenting his or her boss with information and limits. The really responsible, powerful employee will go to the boss and say, "Look, here's what I can do for you that works within the confines of the eight-hour day. If this doesn't seem like enough, we might need to hire another person part-time, or else prioritize my work load differently."

You'd be surprised how well a boss will usually take those kinds of suggestions—suggestions that show you have put time and effort into trying to make the workplace run more smoothly to meet your boss's needs and goals. These contributions are distinctly different from complaining about how inept the boss is behind his back or becoming angry and threatening to his face. Most people respond well to emotionally healthy suggestions.

Employees frequently fear bosses when there is nothing to fear. Your boss is not your parent; you are not a child. Speak with your boss adult to adult, and you can probably come to some agreement. Never—never—get yourself in a stew about a boss, ADD or not. Do your job, be straightforward and respectful, and look out for your own needs.

Ending the Working Relationship

After you've tried everything else, you may need to suggest that your employee or coworker with ADD find more suitable placement—another job. I want to emphasize that this will only be a last resort. He might work hard to overcome his difficulties, his coworkers might accommodate them, or a shift in job responsibilities might accomplish the changes you'd like to see. Still, when all else fails, you may need to counsel him out of a job. Doing this is an art.

Throughout the process, maintain respect for all involved and honor the ADD employee's sense of integrity. Assume he has been willing to do whatever was necessary to learn to accommodate his deficiencies on the job. Also assume that others in the workplace have made reasonable accommodations to his needs.

Yet the person with ADD might not in fact have been willing to work hard to try to overcome the difficult aspects of his ADD. Maybe he had been trying to overcome his difficulties, but his coworkers weren't bending enough to help him succeed. Either way, if the overall work doesn't improve, it may be time for that employee to move on and try something new.

Some jobs require reams of documentation before someone can be let go. Surely, any employer needs to have substantial reasons for letting someone go. With good employee counseling, rather than a power struggle evolving, the transition can usually be made for the best interests of everyone involved.

For your part as the one breaking the bad news, take your time and be thorough every step of the way. Be sure alternate solutions to the workplace problem have been given reasonable chances to work. If the employee still has to be let go, prepare suggestions and opportunities to make the change less traumatic, and ultimately positive for him. Think of job settings where he might be a better fit, and jot down industries or specific companies you think might provide such settings. You may wish to provide the person the opportunity to work with someone in an outplacement or counseling capacity, so check on what would currently be available.

When the time comes to actually have the discussion with the employee, be unshakeable in your resolve to treat him with courtesy and respect. Realistically, if he has a temperament problem or has been truly irresponsible, he may not be able to take the news very well, and it may seem like your preparations, courtesy, and suggestions will not work. Still, you need to act earnestly and caringly.

Begin by summing up everyone's attempts to make a fit for him at the workplace. Note how you and he have both been frustrated when the results were unsatisfactory for everyone.

Next, spell out this employee's strengths. Tell him he deserves to be in a setting that utilizes those strengths.

You might say, "This project [company] can't make the kind of good use of your talents that you deserve. There are better settings for you to work in." Present some of the suggestions you had prepared beforehand.

Finally, tell him specifically when the transition is to be made. Some companies think that once a person is told he is being let go, he needs to pack up that very day; others give four months or more lead time. This decision depends on the individuals involved. If you have a good relationship with the person, you might want him to finish the project at hand, take time off to pursue additional training, or switch to a part-time consulting or contract basis.

On the other hand, you might be a non-ADD employee in an incompatible situation with an ADD boss. You must decide whether you can work with the person or not. If you have tried to get along, do your job, and make accommodations, or if the boss is unwilling to work to improve the situation, you need to consider jumping ship.

But don't act hastily.

Burning your bridges shatters the network you have spent time building. You never know who knows who else nor when or where you could use a good word from a previous boss, even a bad one. Bad-mouthing a boss, no matter how awful the situation might have been, only leads to trouble. Those who don't know the situation may think you're a troublemaker and think less of you. Also, word might get back to the old boss, who will not appreciate your attitude and may find a listening audience for his own viewpoint. Even bad bosses have friends and cronies who like him, and you may need something from one of them sometime.

Furthermore, haste may cheat you of the time you need to make a smooth transition. Your present position, although uncomfortable, can be used as a ramp to launch yourself. Stay in control of your situation. Do as much preplanning or thinking as you can. Get to know yourself and what you want. Think about the kind of boss you'd like to have, or start laying out a plan for self-employment, if this is the time to try that road.

Success in Working with Someone Who Has ADD

It was necessary to use many pages of this book to discuss the difficulties caused by ADD in order to present suggestions and solutions for the workplace issues that confront people with ADD and those who work with us. However, a very important truth is that there are just as many positive aspects to being ADD as negative ones. When people who are ADD do find their fit in the workplace, they are extremely valuable.

I have a fantasy that by the year 2000, people will know how they are wired, and workplace teams will be built to utilize the differences each person brings to the project or job. Equally respected, the skills of all types of people will be properly utilized.

Some such teaming is already happening. Composers and lyricists have formed powerful teams for many years. Computer geniuses and businesspeople have come together to create powerful worldwide companies. Race car drivers and pit crews have produced trips to the winner's circle.

I'd like to share with you four true examples of career success and winning partnerships—partnerships that not only have utilized someone with ADD to advantage but have been possible only *because* of ADD traits.

They call her Cuttie (for Cut-Up), a nickname she acquired at age 3. First her family labeled her, with love and humor; then her teachers continued the tradition; finally, her coworkers called her Cuttie, too, even when she became their boss.

Trained as a teacher, Cuttie's interest in creative dramatics emerged early. After a few years working in the public school system, however, she felt stifled by limitations. She loved working with the kids, so, on a moderately researched impulse, she decided to start her own creative dramatics company.

With charisma, enormous energy, and wonderful, wild ideas, she carved a niche for herself in a big city. Contracting back to the school system, which she had left without burning her bridges, she branched out to contracting to the suburbs and private schools. After a while she ran an after-school program. Then came a summer program, a video, and eventually multimedia creations.

Cuttie hired several teachers who are not ADD to work with her in the areas of drama, art, music, and movement. In an environment of mutual respect, she showed them her strengths and asked for their help in relation to her weaknesses. Cuttie is mostly an Outwardly Expressive ADD person, but she has a bit of perfectionism when it comes to her craft. The Highly Structured part of her ADD helps her in business. She learned early on to hire someone who knew how to handle figures, develop a business plan, and write a proposal.

Because of this partnership, Cuttie has been very successful—while having the time of her life. I promise you, she has brought joy into the lives of the children and families whom she's touched. Her ADD creates magic. Those who work with her know it, admire her, and love her. She in turn respects them, and they are all making a good living because of the special gifts of Cuttie's ADD.

Doc is a pediatrician, and he's ADD. Like most ADD doctors, he has a lot of Highly Structured wiring. Though he has a tendency not to always listen well to those who work for him, he also has a sweet nature. He's never an ogre, so his staff seems to understand that "that's just the way he is" and excuse him. When necessary, they set a limit on him, saying, "You're not listening." When he hears that, he opens his eyes wide and listens attentively—until his mind wanders off on whatever path emerges.

Doc writes poetry, too. That's when his sensitivity really shows. He shares his deep inner feelings in that format, feelings that he can't quite say out loud, face to face with someone. Then there's his clinic program. He opens his doors to the kids and families of people with ADD. He allows his staff to be innovative, does free public education, and recently joined with colleagues to learn more about working with adults who are ADD.

Doc's life has improved quite a bit since he's realized what causes some of his distractibility, overorganization, and impulsivity. Maybe he hasn't accumulated as much money as some of his colleagues, but he's a huge success in my book. His staff appreciates him, and he's making a difference—and it's all because of his ADD.

On a very hot Texas summer afternoon, Bruce can be seen running outside, dropping to the ground to crawl under a car to better hear what an engine is communicating. The car's owner is afraid something big might be wrong. Bruce, upon crawling out, smiles shyly and says, "Oh, it's just a broken nut. I'll have it welded back in a few minutes. Can you wait?" Sure enough, a few minutes later he reappears with a quietly purring car. "No charge," he tells the relieved owner.

Bruce works for a small-town car dealership that serves an entire county in central Texas. Although a high school graduate, he didn't do very well in school because he was distractible, extremely active, and poorly organized. When he was a child, his parents had been told he was hyperactive.

Twenty years ago, Bruce could already fix anything on wheels. Just leave him alone and he'd get the job done. He has always had an intuitive knowledge of engines, and he has *never* been wrong! Fortunately for all of us, he trusts his judgment, and so do his bosses and coworkers.

Starting as a mechanic, Bruce worked his way up, until he made the whole service department hum. He's a little slower using the parts books than his parts man is, but he knows what goes where. It's only copying all the numbers that takes a little extra time.

Bruce's biggest asset to the company and his coworkers might be his attitude. He's nice. He likes what he does. He knows he has a job for life, and he's grateful. Not a great student when young, at first he was afraid that he wouldn't be able to be successful or provide well for the family he hoped to have someday. Now he knows he can; he is thankful, and he shows it.

The final story I'd like to share is autobiographical. It took a long time for me to feel I wasn't a fake. I knew that by a lot of people's standards, I was a success because I had a college degree and two graduate degrees. I knew how much time it took me to get them, though, and how difficult it was, and my grades just weren't that great. In fact, because I had difficulty concentrating, I wasn't able to get a sufficiently high grade on the Graduate Record Exam to get into the graduate school of my choice.

But I did have passion for two things. First, I felt enormous empathy for people and seemed to be able to intuitively know what they needed. Because I wanted to make people's lives better, I chose the field of counseling and stayed in school to earn the credentials that would allow me to help others professionally.

What I never told anyone until many years later, was how I knew what to do while I was in training. I didn't study books on how to do counseling; I just went in a room with someone who was hurting emotionally and kind of played it by ear. I recalled some things that had worked for me when I was the recipient of counseling, and I paid close attention to what seemed to work and what didn't. Years later, I realized that most people communicate what they need if the observer has eyes to see, ears to hear, and a gut-level feeling that can be trusted.

I have built a system inside myself, like the auto mechanic, that is infallible. I didn't know that at first. I kept collecting data and checking to see if I was right. Colleagues and staff learned to trust my way of doing things, too, and they love it when I trust their intuition. My sensitivity comes from my being ADD, though I didn't know that until a short while ago.

Then there was the period of time I was also a radio talk show host and television commentator. Being an Outwardly Expressive ADD person, I became an avid performer over the years. It took a while for that part of me to come to the surface, though, because I was working so hard to survive and trying so hard to be accepted by "the establishment." Maturity did bring freedom, and I found I was an outgoing, at times funny, very verbal woman who definitely loved her audiences.

Because I'm rather strong willed, the people who worked with me either loved me or didn't much like dealing with me. Because I was on a mission of sorts to protect the underdog and tell the truth, I accepted the fact that not everyone would like me. All I could and can do is tell my truth and label it that way.

I have been successful. That success has been because of my ADD.

My second passion has to do with being creative. I forced that part of myself underground for a long time, in the name of seriousness. I've discovered that it sneaked out anyway, surfacing in the form of creative ideas and ways of working with people. It allowed me to consider ADD in adults when authorities were convinced that it went away at puberty. I wasn't afraid to follow a new path, and this creative way of thinking is due to my ADD wiring.

I've learned that many of the working relationships I have are due to my teammates' and coworkers' appreciation of the creativity, enthusiasm, and strong beliefs I have for my missions. All of these traits are due to my ADD, for which I give thanks.

Also because of ADD, I've been blessed to help many people, give hope to more, and experience joy at a level that many people never achieve. And, oh yes, the good news is that being hyperactive, I stay younger than many of my agemates as I get older.

Slow to mature, slow to age, I am enjoying every minute of a fantastic ride on the ADD Express.

11

101 Tips for Managing Your ADD

Information Tips

1. You don't have ADD—you are ADD.
2. ADD is a "flavor," or style, of brain organization that you're born with, grow up with, and die with, so don't let anyone judge you for the way you are.
3. Tell anyone who asks, "ADD is the way I am 'wired.'"
4. You are neither disordered nor deficient, only different—but they are different, too.
5. As many assets as liabilities come from ADD.
6. ADD explains why some things are hard to do while others are easy.
7. Some of the most well-known, talented people throughout history were, or are, ADD.
8. Not everyone with ADD appears the same way. You'll have your own special combination of ADD traits.
9. There is more to you than ADD.

Attitude Tips

10. You've got power when you know how your ADD affects you.

11. Appreciate your ADD, and it will work on your behalf.

12. Know a good thing when you see it, using all the positive attributes your ADD gives you.

13. Cut out judgments of yourself and everyone else who is or isn't ADD. Insist others do the same with you.

14. ADD is not an excuse: it's an explanation.

15. You can be responsible for your ADD.

16. You are valuable as you are, despite what you might have been told.

17. Appreciate and respect differences, your own and others'.

Work Tips

18. You are responsible for adjusting for your ADD without becoming like a non-ADD person.

19. Make a trade with someone to do the tasks that are difficult for you.

20. Tell others about your ADD if you have useful suggestions to share that improve your work or time together.

21. When negotiating, don't stop until a creative solution has been reached in which everyone gets what he needs or wants.

Work Tips for Outwardly Expressive ADD People

22a. Give yourself plenty of room to roam and move about.

23a. Let yourself be expressive.

24a. Watch out that your exuberance doesn't overwhelm others.

25a. When you're excited about something, be careful that you don't get tricked into thinking others can keep up with you.

26a. Leave time to play. You need it.

27a. Make changes, but stay in control of when and how you make them.

28a. Find someone to help you plan and structure your life.

29a. Sometimes listen and learn from others.

30a. Don't be afraid to follow your dreams, even when they are big ones.

31a. Strongly consider going into business for yourself, with clerical and planning support.

Work Tips for Inwardly Directed ADD People

22b. Acknowledge your interests.

23b. Find work settings in which you can utilize your talents and gifts.

24b. Be cautious about getting so immersed in what you love to do that you don't see what's happening around you.

25b. Dream your dreams and believe in them and yourself.

26b. Get help to speak up for what you want.

27b. Be sure to speak up for what you want.

28b. Give yourself the freedom you desire to feel good.

29b. Consider developing partnerships with outgoing people.

30b Strongly consider self-employment, with assistance with paperwork.

31b. Know when to say no.

Work Tips for Highly Structured ADD People

22c. Find ready-made structures to work in that make use of your desire for things to be regular, systematic, and just so.

23c. Be sure you work around people and in a setting that reflect your values.

24c. Give yourself permission to relax as much as you can stand.

25c. Be sure to apply your desire for perfectionism only to yourself—not to others.

26c. Let go of judgments, seeing differences between people and their abilities as just that: differences.

27c. Mind your own business, not others'.

28c. Be sure to treat or pamper yourself for jobs well done.

29c. Take responsibility for half of every problem you are involved with.

30c. Keep criticism to a minimum.

31c. Be kind to yourself.

Behavioral Tips

32. Tell the truth, except on the rare occasions when the person listening can't handle it.

33. When you act impulsively or lose your temper, figure out what you were feeling immediately beforehand.

34. Give yourself permission to protect your sensitive self, but seek ways that won't hurt you in the process; don't impulsively quitting your job.

35. Don't believe anyone who tells you you're too sensitive.

36. Use your sensitivity to advantage, trusting what you feel, see, and hear. Your intuition will be your greatest tool.

37. Be true to the way you learn. If you're a kinesthetic learner, ask people to show you how to do things, not tell you.

38. Add humor in the right places, but know when to turn it off.

39. Get help with any addictions, and don't fool yourself into thinking they don't make a difference.

40. Stop doing what you "should" do. Instead do what you want to do and take responsibility for the results.

Organizational Tips

41. Know which type or types of ADD you are and note how it affects your sense of time.

42. Relieve others from the effects of your poor time sense. Go it alone until you have time under control.

43. Reward yourself for good time management.

44. Break large tasks down into manageable bits.

45. If you're messy but you know where things are, don't change— unless you're driving someone else crazy. Then negotiate.

46. Get help with paperwork as needed: work on it with someone else, or turn it over to someone else completely.

47. Organize things any way you like that works for you. There's no one right way.

48. Decide whether you do better sticking to a project until it's done or breaking it up into miniprojects. Give yourself rewards each step of the way.

49. Realize there's nothing sacred about being well organized.

Communication Tips

50. Remember, people are rarely let go from a job because they lack technical skills; it's usually because of poor communication.

51. Speak up for what you want or need to do your job efficiently or better.

52. Watch out for assumptions on your part and on the part of others.

53. Listen to others.

54. Warn people you work with that you sometimes (or often) say, "Uh-huh," without really hear what they've asked you or said.

55. You have just as much of value to say as anyone else. Say it.

56. Work on dialoguing back and forth with others and negotiating points of view.

57. Try to understand another's point of view, even though you don't agree with it.

58. Learn to say no and set other limits on people and situations.

Relationship Tips

59. All healthy relationships are based on mutual respect. Start by respecting yourself.

60. Being different doesn't mean you're wrong or bad. Apply this to yourself and others.

61. Concentrate on what's valuable about another person, rather than what you don't like.

62. Realize that all people have strengths and weaknesses. No one is intrinsically better or less adequate than any other person, only different.

63. When you don't agree with another person, ask for his or her perspective on the situation, rather than accusing him or her.

64. Strive for consensus—where everyone wins when resolving differences—rather than trying to win.

65. If you don't understand office politics, ask a trusted colleague or coworker to explain them to you.

66. The world needs teams of people who know how to respect and honor one another.

67. Be clear with coworkers, separating your personal feelings from you work relationships.

68. Treat others as you would like to be treated.

69. Treat yourself as well as you treat others.

70. Show respect for everyone.

Stress Management Tips

71. No job is as important as the well-being of the person in it.

72. Stop beating up on yourself because you do things differently from others.

73. You must fit any job you are in to avoid stress.

74. Job-related stress shows itself physically, mentally, and emotionally. Know the signs and watch for them.

75. Determine whether your stress is temporary or chronic. Cope with temporary stress, make changes in relation to chronic stress.

76. Prevent stress from building up by identifying sources of stress.

77. Learn and use stress reduction techniques regularly.

78. Be sure that your recreation is stress free.

79. Treat stress conditions seriously. Don't keep pushing yourself through the symptoms; change your way of life.

Employment Tips

80. Make sure your work reflects your talents and strengths, rather than your liabilities.

81. Be clear about the natural you—who you are, what you like, what you value, and your goals in life.

82. Do not feel guilty about anything that you like or about your way of doing things.

83. Come out of the closet and show others who you truly are.

84. Be sure to update your identity now that you know that you are ADD.

85. Try new things in order to learn what you like.

86. Do what you like. Don't do what you don't like.

87. If you need to change the way you've been doing things, change. Take your lumps from having gone down a wrong path and go on, thankful that you've awakened.

88. Start today to make any changes you want.

89. If you can dream it, you can do it. You may only need to learn to do, or to change the way you go about doing, what you dream about.

When-You-Need-a-Lift Tips

90. You are lucky you are ADD!

91. ADD people are naturally creative, compassionate, energetic people who make the world a more joyous place in which to live.

92. Lots of us are around; you are not alone.

93. Everyone has innate talents and gifts that the world and the people in it need. That includes you.

94. People who are ADD are as intelligent as anyone else.

95. Life may have been tough up until now, but today is the day to look at yourself in a new light. See a winner? I do.

96. You can be ADD and be successful.

97. When you use your ADD to advantage, you take power into your own hands.

98. You can learn anything, as long as you go about learning it in your own way.

99. You can heal your past hurts and use your experience to help others. You are needed.

100. You are valuable.

101. I'm glad you were born. The world is a better place because of you.

Appendix

The Rehabilitation Act of 1973, relating to the activities of the federal government and entities receiving federal assistance, considered "Specific Learning Disabilities" an impairment. The Americans with Disabilities Act (ADA) of 1990 relates to the activites of state and local governments, programs conducted for state and local governments, and entities in the private sector. Again "Specific Learning Disabilities" was recognized as a category of impairment.

Attention deficit disorder is listed as one of the "Specific Learning Disabilities." Information about ADA can be obtained from the following sources:

The Rebus Institute
1499 Bayshore Boulevard
Suite 146
Burlingame, CA 94010
(415) 697–7424

Southwest Disability and Business
  Technical Assistance Center
2323 South Shepherd, Suite 1000
Houston, TX 77019
Voice/TTY: (800) 949–4232

United States Department of
  Justice
Office of Americans with
  Disabilities Act
Civil Rights Division
P.O. Box 66118
Washington, D.C. 20035
(800) 514–0301 (voice);
(800) 514–0383 (TDD)

United States Equal Employment
  Opportunity Commission
P.O. Box 12549
Cincinnati, OH 45212–0549
(800) 669–3362 (voice);
(800) 800–3302 (TDD)
Job Accommodation Network
(800) 526–7234 (voice);
(800) 526–7234 (TDD)

Index

A

Accidents, stress in, 141

Accountant, need for, 188

Addictive behavior in ADD, 32–35

Affirmation, asking directly for, 67

Alcohol, 32

Alcoholism, 33–37

American Psychiatric Association's Diagnostic and Statistical Manual, on classification of ADD, 5

Americans with Disabilities Act (ADA) (1990), 86, 114, 218

Anger, 38

as cover up emotion, 197

Anxiety, and stress, 142

Appetite, loss or increase of, and stress, 141

Assignments, talking your way through, 79

Attention, characteristics, of problems with, 198

Attention deficit disorder (ADD), 211. *See also* Highly structured ADD; Inwardly directed ADD; Outwardly expressive ADD

and addictive behaviors, 32–35

in adults, 3–4, 161–62

alternative view of, 5–8

appropriate model for, 6

attitude tips for, 212

authority problems related to, 116–17

behavioral tips for, 214

characteristics of person with, 4–5

common behaviors attributed to, 11–12

communication tips for, 215

and eating habits, 147–48

employment tips for, 216–17

information tips for managing, 211

making accommodations for, 1–4, 7–8

organizational tips for, 214

recognizing, in workplace, 36

relationship tips for, 215–16

stress management tips for, 216

telling coworker about, 87–89

time-related conflicts

between non-ADD coworkers and, 45–46

between people with different types of, 44–45

types of, 8–9

and different types of behavior, 28–32

when-you-need-a-lift tips for, 217

in workplace, 6–7, 191–210

tips for, 212–13

Attitude tips for managing ADD, 212

Auditory aids, and time management, 47

Authority issues, related to the ADD employee, 116–17

Awareness, multiple-track, 26–27